Inflammation

Anti-Inflammatory Diet

Overcome Inflammation Naturally Without Taking Medication

Introduction

<u>Put an end to inflammation naturally by implementing the natural strategies that this book discusses.</u>

What do you think about when someone mentions inflammation? Does the picture of a swollen leg or any other body part after an accident come to mind at the mention of inflammation?

Well, while this is a form of inflammation, it is really harmless even when it comes with a lot of pain. In fact, the body is doing you a favor at the time when it is hurting so bad-you just might not understand it at the time. You need not be afraid of this painful inflammation that comes after an injury or disease. However, **<u>there is a type of inflammation that you need to be afraid of i.e. the type that is not as painful, at least in the beginning</u>**!

Your body might be inflamed due to various reasons including toxins, autoimmune diseases, excessive weight, and other reasons. And when this happens, you will probably not experience any pain. However, **<u>just because you don't experience pain doesn't mean that you are just fine;</u>**

in fact, the situation might be getting worse with every passing day.

This **signifies that you have chronic inflammation, which needs to be addressed fast.**

The question you may have is; **what are the risks of such an inflammation?** Well, for starters, inflammation **can make it almost impossible for you to lose weight so unless you fix it**, you can **kiss goodbye any hopes of losing weight unless you opt for invasive weight loss methods.**

It can also set the stage for the development of a wide array of other health conditions among them cancers, arthritis, diabetes, hypertension and many others. Obviously, you really don't want that for yourself!

So what do you do?

The best solution for this problem is through diet.

Well, lucky for you, this book will show you how to fight inflammation through diet.

<u>It will help you to understand:</u>

- How inflammation develops

- **The causes, the risks**

- The foods you should take to fight inflammation

- **The foods you should avoid in your journey to fighting inflammation**

- Over 40 delicious anti-inflammatory diet recipes

- **Tips that will hold you by the hand on your journey to fighting inflammation**

- And much, much more!

If you are ready to stop inflammation in its tracks before it causes severe damages and makes your life unbearable, let's get started.

You won't regret it!

I hope you enjoy it!

PS: I'd like your feedback. If you are happy with this book, please <u>leave a review on Amazon</u>.

Table of Contents

Breakfast Recipes _______________________ 136

Lunch Recipes ________________________ 156

Understanding Inflammation

An anti-inflammatory diet is a collection of foods, which are capable of fighting chronic inflammation in your body. But what exactly is chronic inflammation? To help you understand chronic inflammation, you need to understand inflammation first. Inflammation is the first response that your immune system has towards any of your body injuries with the intention of healing the affected area. It is actually the way the body protects itself from viruses, bacteria, and various other microbes in order to accelerate healing. However, there are instances when the body might have an inflammatory response even when the situation does not pose any threat to the body. When this happens, especially over a prolonged period, this can result to cell and tissue damage. There are two forms of inflammation i.e. acute inflammation and chronic inflammation.

1. Acute inflammation

When an injury occurs, in your body an inflammatory response is launched with an army of white blood cells, which are sent straight to the scene to provide assistance. During this process, three things happen:

- The small branches of your arteries (arterioles) dilate resulting to increased blood flow.

- The capillaries, which supply blood to the injured region, become more permeable allowing blood proteins and fluids to easily move between the cells.

- Neutrophils (it's a white blood cell full of tiny sacs that contain enzymes responsible for digesting microorganisms) and Macrophages (the white blood cells responsible for ingesting foreign materials) move from the capillaries and into the spaces between the cells.

Those are the three major cells that take up the responsibility of protecting us from bacterial infections. When the three things above happen, your body responds in the following ways:

Signs of acute inflammation

- Redness – this results from the unusual extra blood in the capillaries.

- Swelling – as a result of accumulated fluids

- Pain – the chemicals that are released to stimulate nerve endings are very sensitive and that's why the inflamed area is painful particularly when touched.

- Heat- the excessive blood in the inflamed area experiences a hot sensation.

Acute inflammation is an outstanding process that is good for optimum health. It might not look like it on the swollen or reddish surface but it is actually all part of making the affected area better.

As you can notice, the layman's understanding of inflammation is acute inflammation. This is not the only form of inflammation.

2. Chronic inflammation

While inflammation might be good for you, the truth is that not all types of inflammations are good for you. This 'bad' type of inflammation is referred to as chronic inflammation. When the body's inflammatory response is not caused by an injury, there is a high likelihood you might be suffering from chronic inflammation.

How does this occur? As we have discussed, inflammation is supposed to be a first response reaction to offering assistance for an injury after which the inflammatory response dies down to give way to other healing processes. When the inflammation goes against this principal and overstays its welcome in the affected area, it results to your body functioning as if it is constantly under attack. This in turn means that there is a likelihood that your white blood cells keep on existing in one area in a permanent activation mode. Soon, your immune system becomes exhausted and has no energy left to deploy your white blood cells to deal with other illnesses such as cancer cells, bacterial infections and viruses. And when this happens, you are likely to start noticing any of the following symptoms:

Symptoms of chronic inflammation

- Diarrhea

- Dry eyes

- Congestion

- Stiffness of joints and muscles

- Skin outbreaks

- Body aches and severe pains

- Swelling

- Loss of joint function

- Headaches

- Fever, chills, fatigue and loss of energy

- In critical conditions, you might experience damage of your cartilage or suffer from various autoimmune diseases like arthritis, cancer, diabetes and many others (I will show you the link between these diseases and inflammation).

Next, we will be discussing how inflammation begins along with the different diseases that come with inflammation.

Where Does Chronic Inflammation Begin?

Chronic inflammation begins in your gut and I am going to dedicate this chapter to show you how this happens. Your gut is a huge semi porous lining, which fluctuates in response to the variety of chemicals that come into contact with it. For example, if your cortisol is high as a result of stress or your thyroid hormone levels are changing from time to time, your intestinal lining will change to become extra permeable. Poor gut health has actually been shown to be closely related to suppressed thyroid function.

This paves way for toxins, yeast, bacteria, viruses, and undigested foods to pass through your intestines and get into your bloodstream. What I have just described is called leaky gut syndrome (LGS).

When your intestinal lining is repetitively damaged, your microvilli become crippled and unable to do their job, which is processing and utilizing nutrients with some enzymes that are essential for proper digestion. Ultimately, this weakens your digestive system resulting to poor absorption of nutrients. As exposure continues, your body reacts by initiating attacks on the foreign invaders and this ultimately results to inflammation and allergic reactions.

Unlike acute inflammation, which is a healthy process, this form of inflammation is harmful and can even cause different health complications. When this is coupled with the fact that such reactions often make the body to keep on producing white blood cells to fight any of the 'foreign bodies' that find their way into the bloodstream, this can result to inflammatory triggers around the body. When this happens for a long time, it might negatively affect your organs, joints, muscles, connective tissues, and nerves. This can manifest in the form of various health complications that we will discuss next. This is what is referred to as an autoimmune response. Autoimmune diseases are illnesses caused by your own body defense system attacking your tissues instead of viruses, germs and other foreign substances.

Diseases Associated With Inflammation

Here are some few health complications that are often associated with inflammation:

Arthritis: The attack from your own defensive system causes stiffness, joint damage, and pain. If you have

Psoriasis, this is associated with inflammation of the skin and the tissues that surround different joints. On the other hand, if you suffer from Ankylosing spondylitis, this one is associated with the inflammation of ligaments, muscles, vertebrae and sacroiliac joints (where the hips and spine meet). Additionally, if you suffer from rheumatoid arthritis, you are likely to suffer from inflammation of joints and the tissues that surround joints. These three types of arthritis can affect the entire body if not addressed early.

Crohn's disease: This is a condition that is caused by inflammation in the gut. The most common symptoms are abdominal pain, diarrhea, and nausea.

Lupus: This is inflammation in the lungs, kidney, skin, and joints.

Fibromyalgia: This condition causes pain in different parts of your body. It is frequently related to other autoimmune disorders like lupus and rheumatoid arthritis.

Celiac diseases: In this case, you experience inflammation of inner lining of your small intestines.

Diabetes*:* Type-2-diabetes has been widely known to skyrocket when a person is obese. Inflammation, obesity, and diabetes are all connected by a protein called cytokines, a protein produced by fat cells to control the level of inflammation; the body normally produces cytokines to control inflammatory responses. However, if these cytokines are produced in excessive or uncontrolled amounts, this can result to destructive inflammatory response. In short, the more the fat your body has, the more the inflammation. Ultimately, this results to excessive circulation of cytokines, which obstructs the ability of the body to control the production of insulin in the body. Type 2 diabetes is associated with high levels of cytokines, which often cause chronic inflammation. The consistently high levels of blood sugar can injure your blood vessels resulting to irritations and plaques, which usually break down and then spread throughout the body to cause cell damage. Actually, the anti-inflammatory response usually causes plaques to rapture resulting to damage to tissues and body organs.

Heart disease: In the past, research showed that heart diseases such as heart attacks and stroke were caused by sticky plaque that stuck on the smooth artery walls. This caused the artery walls to narrow resulting to a blood clot that could block the opening and cause a heart attack. Recent research has discovered that their previous theory was not entirely true. They have now discovered that heart attack stems from chronic inflammation. Let me expound further; medical experts have found out that the artery is not a smooth pipe; it is just a multilayered and dynamic structure of a tissue, which absorbs bad cholesterol originally from the blood stream but instead of clotting, it forms a blister. The body then triggers an inflammatory reaction, which causes the artery to swell under the nervous tension, which blocks blood flow to the heart. You get a heart attack after the blister goes deep in the artery tissue and is covered by a scab-like plaque, which bursts and wrecks the artery.

Cancer: Recent research has shown that inflammation has been playing either a leading role or a supportive role in several common types of cancer like stomach, breast, lung and colon cancer. Colon cancer is a perfect example of a cancer that preys on inflammation. Inflammation sets up the stage for colon cancer by letting free radicals to thrive in the intestines. However, please note that chronic inflammation cannot spark cancer alone but it can create a comfortable place for cancer to prosper in.

Whenever a tumor develops within the cells, this in turn obstructs the cells from oxygen and nutrients making the tumors to grow even bigger. The cancerous cells in turn produce a chemical, which actually causes macrophages and granulocytes immune system cells to infiltrate the tumor after which the cells secrete cytokines, which in turn triggers inflammatory response. Any free radicals that arise from your diet and the chemical reactions in the body can actually split the tumor and cause severe damage to the DNA.

Obesity or weight gain: Inflammation has a profound effect on whether or not you will gain weight. For starters, inflammation affects the functioning of the hormone leptin, the satiety hormone. Leptin is also very important given that it determines the amount of body fat through controlling body fat and appetite. But when you have chronic inflammation, your brain's ability to detect messages from the leptin hormone is impaired, which means that you might not tell when you have had enough food. As a result, you end up taking more calories than necessary resulting to weight gain. As such, the best solution for improving the responsiveness of your brain to leptin is fixing inflammation.

How To Fight Inflammation Naturally

As you have already seen in the previous chapter, inflammation is a health risk, which needs to be stopped. For you to do that, you can use different methods to make this possible. If you want to prevent or reduce inflammation naturally, you need to first learn how to listen to your body. It will help you know what catalyzes your inflammatory responses and what does the opposite. We will discuss different methods through which you can fight inflammation. The first thing we will start with is diet, as diet is also one of the biggest inflammation triggers.

Diet

An anti-inflammatory diet is based on eating foods that prevent inflammatory reactions while ditching those that cause it. You do this through adapting a healthier diet that comprises of less processed foods, no deep-fried foods, no added sugars, low in fats and high in vegetables, fruits and whole grains. Such a diet is also of low-fat, nonfat dairy foods and of high omega 3 fatty acids, which help protect you from developing chronic inflammatory diseases. Such a diet recommends a daily intake of about 2000 to 3000 calories, which primarily depends on your activity level, your body size and gender of course. You may even choose to have 40 to 50 percent of your calories from low carb foods, 20 to 30 percent from protein rich foods and a further 30 percent from healthy fats. If need be, throw in some dark chocolate, green tea and a few spices to make the diet as delicious as possible.

Needless to say, you do not have to count calories in this diet plan as far as you balance your macronutrients- i.e. protein, carbs and fats. Here are a few guidelines you need to observe when choosing a suitable anti-inflammatory diet plan:

1. Eat organic and locally grown fruits and veggies, preferably from your local market for the freshest produce. Such ingredients are less likely to be contaminated with inflammatory substances such as artificial sugars, added salts, chemical-based preservatives or gluten.

2. It's recommended that you ensure that at least half or up to two-thirds of your calories comes from non-starchy veggies as these are rich in disease-fighting antioxidants and fiber that helps balance your gut.

3. Reduce intake of red meat, and ensure you only choose organic varieties of fish, turkey and chicken. Also, avoid

processed meats that are likely to have additives or other inflammatory substances such as those with added sodium nitrite.

4. Concerning fish, opt for herring, mackerel, salmon and anchovies as they have the highest amounts of omega 3 fatty acids that fight inflammation and lowest amounts of mercury, the toxic metal. Alternatively, you can take 1000mg of omega 3 supplements per day.

5. Add in whole grains and organic beans to your diet through various soups and stews you like as these are packed with nutrients and are high in fiber. On top of boosting digestion, fiber also helps reduce your cholesterol levels. Try out millet, brown rice, quinoa and unbleached barley.

6. Limit intake of saturated fats such as vegetable oils and butter and totally avoid those high in inflammatory omega 6 fatty acids such as corn oil and safflower. Only choose oils such as olive oil, walnut oil and avocado as these are not as inflammatory as compared to margarine. Healthy oils can lower total cholesterol and triglyceride levels in your blood plasma, which are linked to heart diseases and other cardio-vascular problems.

7. Reduce or completely ditch sugar and other sweet foods such as honey, fruit juices and most fast foods. Based on a 2005 study , eating a high sugar diet for about 10 weeks can greatly increase blood levels of inflammatory *haptoglobin* that is linked to obesity, stroke, heart attack and diabetes.

8. Avoid white flour-based products such as tortillas, breads and grain crackers and instead take moderate amounts of whole grain-based flours and food varieties such as burger wheat, brown rice and quinoa. Be aware that even whole grain-based flour may still pose a threat for you as far as inflammation is concerned especially if having metabolic syndrome such as diabetes or if insulin resistant.

9. Add spices such as turmeric, rosemary and ginger to your foods as they help reduce inflammation.

While you may find it hard to make such drastic changes in your dieting, you need to appreciate the fact that anti-inflammatory diet is the only sure way to keep of diseases and prolong your life. Healthy diet will reduce chronic pain, reduce risk of cancer and heart attack and make you feel stronger each and every day. Better still, these foods are very beneficial to your health and your general lifestyle on top of preventing or chronic fighting inflammation. Here are the most likely benefits you get with an anti-inflammatory diet:

Why Diet? The Major Benefits of Following An Anti-inflammatory Diet

Foods such as fruits, vegetables, whole grains and nuts are rich in fiber, folate, magnesium and potassium, vitamin A and other antioxidants that promote your general health. Such properties help in the fight against inflammation-related diseases such as cancer, diabetes and the heart disease.

Apart from that, let's see top 5 benefits you get from switching to anti-inflammatory diet:

1. Accelerated Weight loss

Whole foods such as nuts, legumes, fatty fish, whole grains, veggies, fruits, and lean meats do not add unnecessary calories to the body. These foods offer nutrients that support healthy cell function and accelerated metabolism to burn down fat. By following an anti-inflammatory diet, you can lose weight fast within few weeks, especially with moderate exercise routines like walking and occasional jogging. This diet is also rich in satiating foods, which help reduce appetite and unhealthy snacking. Frequent hunger can affect you as a beginner and thus make it harder for you strictly follow the diet.

This dieting lifestyle also incorporates a sufficient amount of healthy fats like olive and coconut oil that promote satiety, boost appetite and curb unnecessary cravings. You also eat ample veggies, which boost satiety, and healthy fruits that increase fiber content. Fiber is important in absorbing the water and takes up much space into the stomach; to help fight hunger or cravings. Whole foods that are rich in fiber include beans, oatmeal and bran cereal. The recommended amount of fiber per day is 25-35 grams, so you should boost your fiber content by more of these foods.

2. Boosts Your Health

Healthy and unprocessed foods can strengthen your immune system and thus minimize risk for hypertension, stroke or the heart disease. For instance, fruits and veggies are rich in vitamin C, which strengthens the blood vessels. Dark green veggies provide you with antioxidants and phytonutrients, which neutralize free radicals that bring diseases like cancer. Yoghurt, ferments foods, fruits and veggies have good bacteria or probiotics help restore gut health and immunity.

Also, healthy fats from olive oil, avocados and nuts can lower blood cholesterol to maintain healthier heart.

3. Boosts Your Mood

Lean proteins from fish and poultry, fruits and veggies help balance your energy level, tone your muscles, give more nutrients and allow you think more clearly. The vitamin B-complex found in fruits and veggies triggers production of dopamine, a hormone that brings happiness and fights stress. Lean protein foods are rich in omega 3 fatty acids, vitamin E and antioxidants that lower cortisol or stress hormone and thus boost your mood.

To get omega 3 fatty acids, go for cold water fish like tuna and salmon, and nuts like almonds and walnuts to benefit from antioxidants like vitamin E that fight diseases. Also eat dark-skinned veggies like bell pepper, eggplant, beets, broccoli, spinach and kales have vitamins and other brain-enhancing nutrients. Similarly, eat plenty of fruits like berries, grapes, prunes, cherries and raisins as these have high quality antioxidants that protect your brain cells.

4. Energizes You

An anti-inflammatory dieting regimen comprises of fruits and veggies, which supply B-complex vitamins and iron, nutrients which facilitate energy or fuel access in the body. Whole foods such as beans and other legumes are also rich in fiber and proteins and also offer a more consistent and steady source of energy. On the other hand, processed carbs such as sweets or refined grains often cause a spike into your blood sugar and trigger cravings and unnecessary eating. Worse still, processed foods have low nutritional value and thus cannot be efficiently utilized to generate energy for cells.

To improve your energy supply, eat protein and fiber-rich foods as these facilitate slow and steady release of calories. You can eat cottage cheese with veggies or hummus, apple slices with peanut butter, oatmeal with fruit, cheese with crackers and yogurt with fruit.

5. Enable You Sleep

Sleep doesn't come as naturally as you might think. In fact, factors such as diet, stress, diseases and other external factors can affect your sleeping patterns. It even gets worse particularly if you suffer from conditions such as rheumatoid arthritis. That notwithstanding, sleep is a vital requirement. Getting 7-9 hours of sleep is vital, as it gives the body sufficient time to build and repair muscle and to establish muscle memory from a workout or project. Restful sleep also helps reduce reaction time to stimuli, sharpens your focus and increases energy levels especially upon waking

Anti-inflammatory diet comprises of whole foods like fruits and veggies which are rich in minerals like magnesium and iron as well as vitamins A; B-complex, E and K. These nutrients help calm your nervous system and also create a hormonal response that promotes good sleep. These minerals work on your brain to facilitate faster and restful sleep, and can also help you achieve longer periods of sleeping. To improve your sleep patterns or enhance a more restful sleep, eat more veggies, fruits and nuts.

In order to achieve these benefits, you need to strictly follow inflammation-fighting diet by only buying foods that are approved as per the diet. You need to avoid refined carbs, foods with added sugars, saturated fats and junk foods that often cause obesity and chronic diseases. However, you may need to check with your doctor before trying out a new dieting lifestyle to avoid any unforeseen problems.

To get you started in your new dieting lifestyle, let's discuss foods to choose from and those to keep away from:

Foods That Have Anti-Inflammatory Properties

Incorporating foods rich in anti-inflammatory properties in your diet is very effective when it comes to fighting inflammation. Let us now look at the different foods and herbs that have anti-inflammatory properties.

1. Foods That Fight Inflammation

As we have seen in the previous chapters, inflammation can still persist in your body long after your injury has been treated. This means we need to have constant solution of dealing with inflammation in our bodies. One of the most effective ways of dealing with inflammation is through foods, which are rich in anti-inflammatory properties. Below are some of the foods you should take to fight inflammation:

Soy

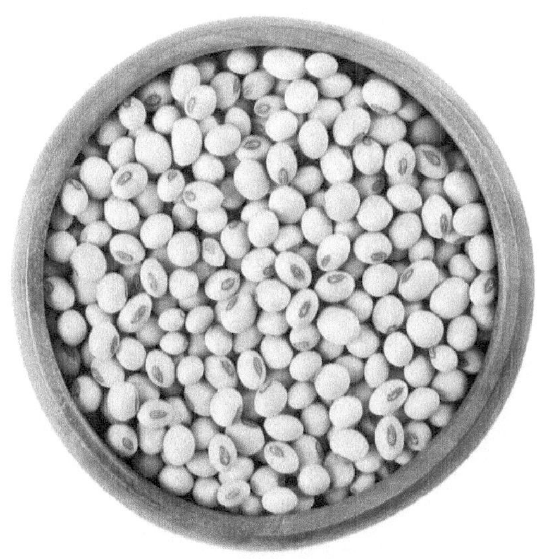

Soy has isoflavones, a substance, which usually works just like estrogen in controlling your mood. It can also lower the rate of inflammation, improve your bone structure, and even restore your heart health. Take soymilk, tofu or boiled soybeans but don't buy processed soy products.

Coconut/ coconut oil

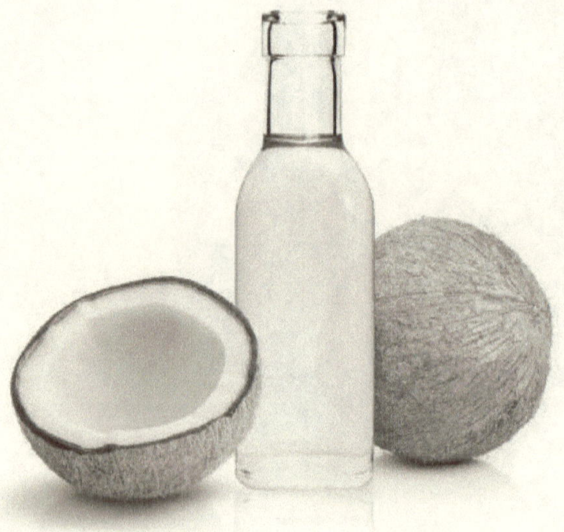

Caprilic and lauric are the medium chain triglycerides, which give both the coconut and its oil strong anti-inflammatory properties. The great thing about coconut oil is that you can use it both topically and internally to fight inflammation. The medium chain triglycerides have anti-microbial properties, which can be very helpful in fighting inflammation.

Seaweeds

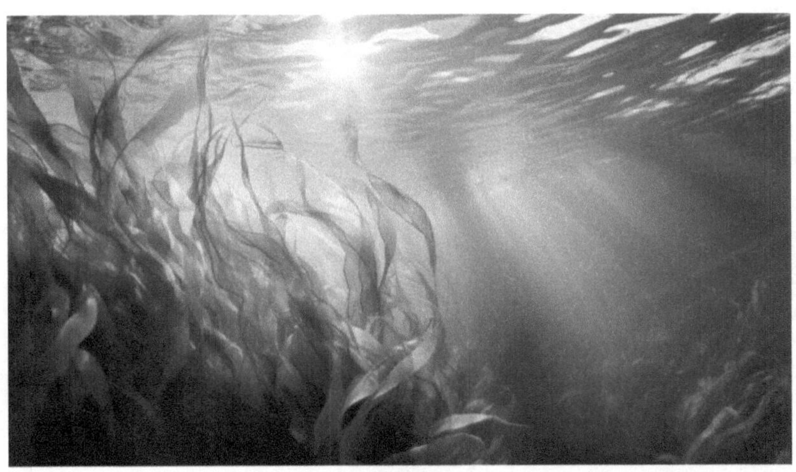

Seaweeds are not only nutritious, they are also highly alkaline, a property, which helps them to sooth the body and fight inflammation. The alkalinity also helps to balance your hormones, remove toxins out of your body, and offer protection from radiation.

Turnips

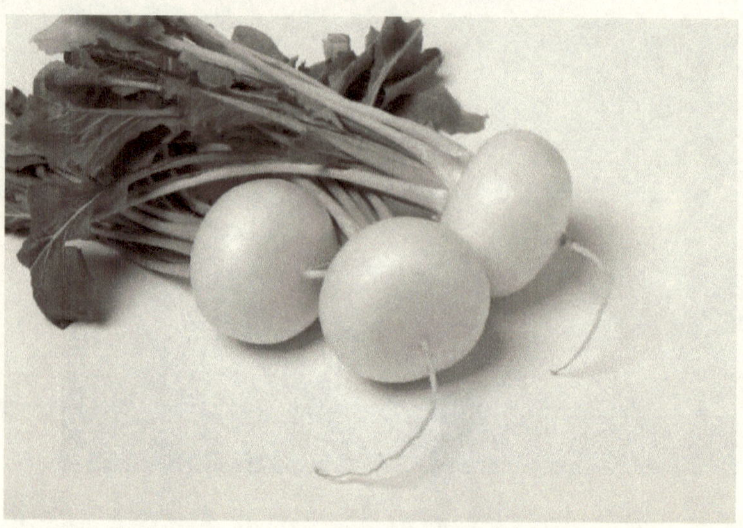

This one is high in omega 3 fatty acids, vitamin C, and vitamin K all of which have anti-inflammatory properties.

Shellfish

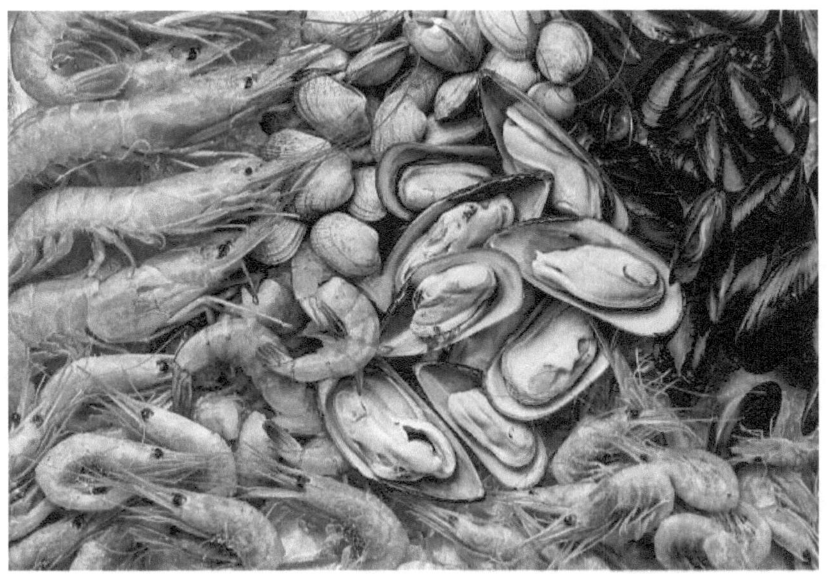

This has a component referred to as astaxanthin, an anti-inflammatory substance, which has been proven to heal joint pain. You should eat lots of shell fish like scallops, shrimp and oysters. However, ensure to take these in moderation given that they are high in cholesterol content.

Leafy Green vegetables

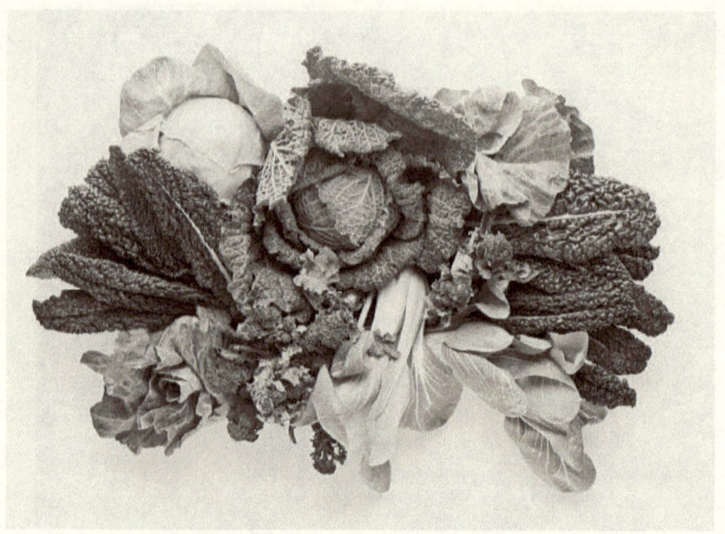

Green veggies have a compound, which is called chlorophyll. Chlorophyll has an amazing alkaline effect, which is very helpful in fighting inflammation. Additionally, green veggies are high in vitamin E, calcium, and iron all of which are very helpful in fighting inflammation. For instance, vitamin E helps reduce the amount of cytokines in the body. Green veggies also have high levels of phytochemicals and minerals all of which help in fighting inflammation, weight gain and other complications. Regular consumption of leafy green vegetables is highly recommended for both the people who suffer from inflammation and those who don't. Some examples of good veggies to consume are romaine, kale, swiss chard, collard greens, red leaf lettuce, spinach and green leaf lettuce. Take soft greens like lettuces if you have a sensitive gut.

Dark green veggies

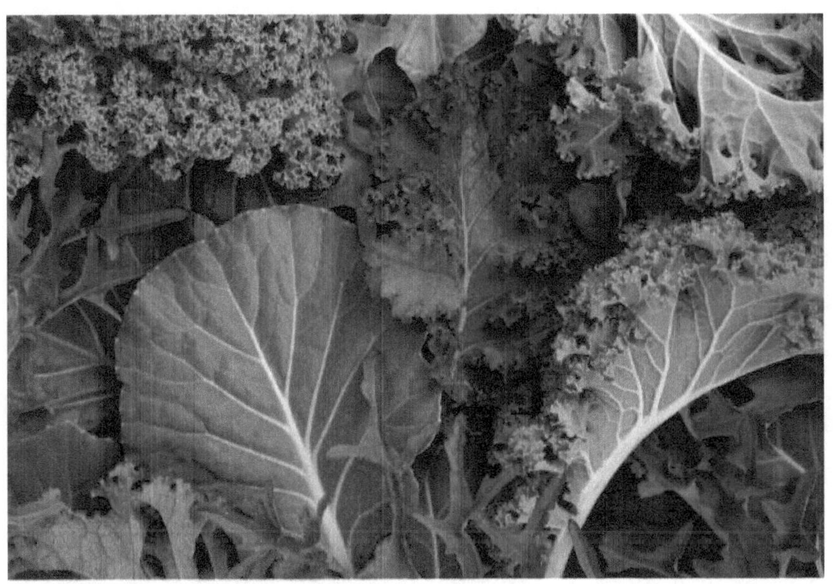

Just like leafy green veggies, dark green veggies are rich in chlorophyll, which, as we have discussed fights inflammation. Examples of dark green veggies are broccoli, zucchini, cucumber, and celery.

Omega 3 fatty acid rich foods

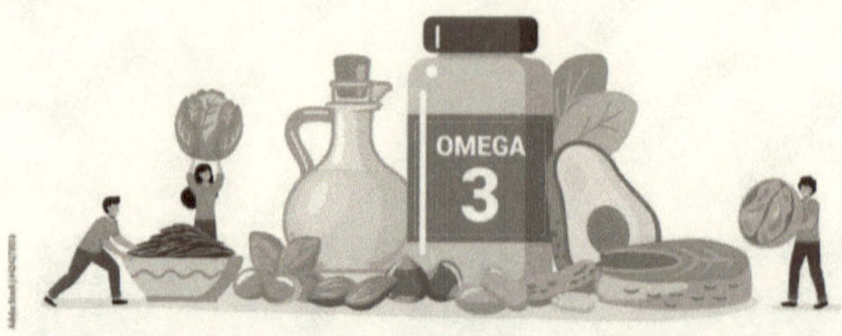

The omega 3 rich foods have the ability to stop the inflammatory process by blocking the prostaglandin pathways (which manufactures inflammation) and supports the prostaglandin pathways that trim down inflammation. You should definitely take more omega 3 fatty acid rich foods like avocados, olives, hemp seeds, walnuts and chia seeds. You should also take fish since it is high in omega 3 fatty acids, which ultimately help counter the effects of autoimmune diseases. In this case, you should take more of boiled or baked tuna, salmon, sardines, and mackerel since they are high in omega 3 fatty acids. In so doing, you reduce the risk of heart attack by about 23% if you avoid dried or salted fish.

I will discuss some of the specific omega 3 fatty acid rich foods, as these have a lot more to offer than just omega 3 fatty acids.

Salmon

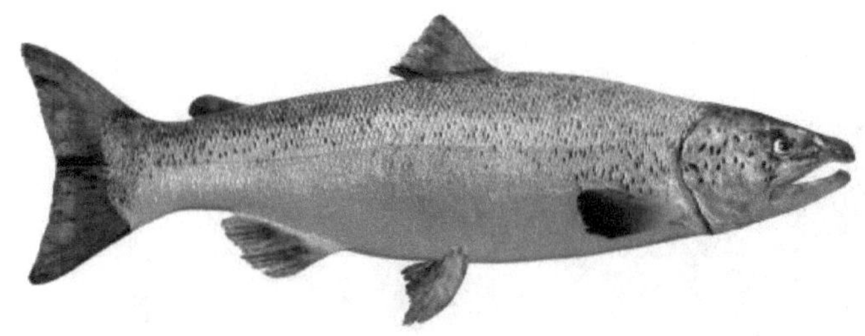

This fatty fish is a good source of omega 3 fatty acids that are a powerhouse in terms of fighting inflammatory diseases. Based on studies, eating salmon regularly can offer significant relief from chronic diseases and greatly reduce need for pharmaceutical medications. Your brain is mostly concentrated with omega 3 fatty acids, which research shows help boost behavioral function, brain memory and its function. To maintain a healthy brain, ensure that you supplement with cold water fish or wild-caught, salmon which has more nutrients compared to farmed fish.

Chia Seeds

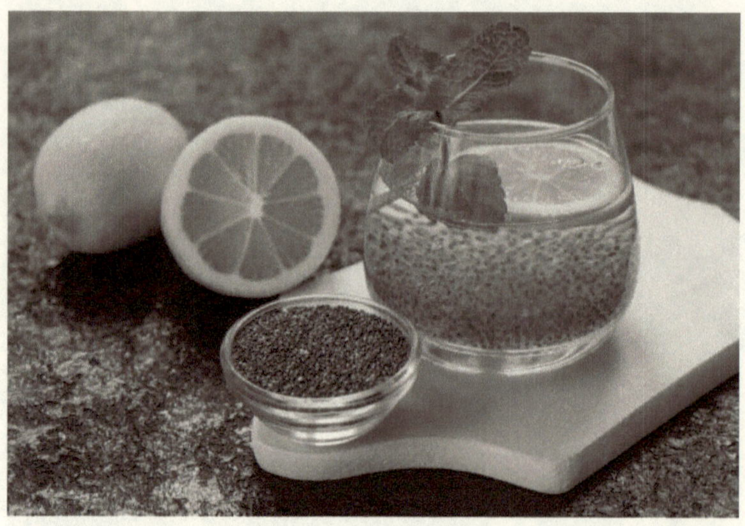

Seeds such as chia are rich in both omega 3 and omega 6 fatty acids whose concurrence has been proven to balance each other in the body. Chia seeds are also rich in minerals such as magnesium, iron and vitamins A, B and E, along with essential fatty acids such as linoleic and alpha-linolenic acids. These phytonutrients help regulate cholesterol, prevent inflammation and boost heart health. Chia seeds also reverse oxidative stress thereby helping reduce risk of getting atherosclerosis.

Flaxseeds

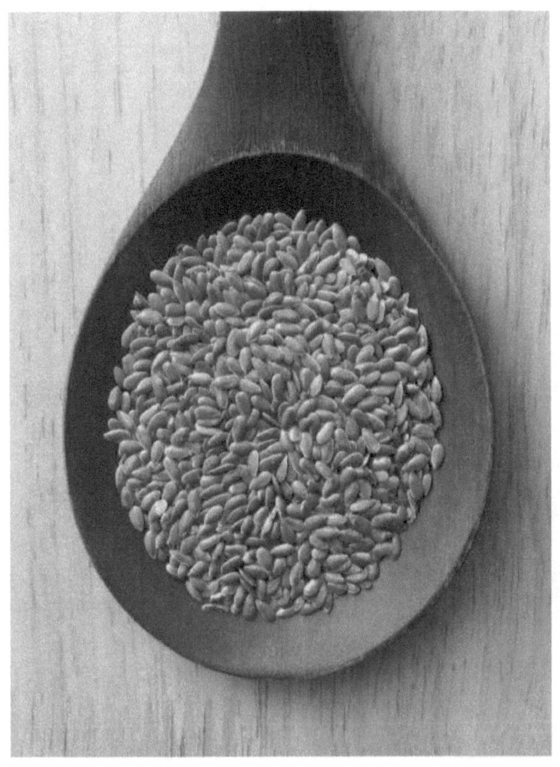

Another seed to embrace is flaxseed that is packed with omega 3 fatty acids and powerful anti-oxidants. It has fiber-related polyphenols called *lignans* that offer anti-oxidant benefits among them proper cellular health, hormonal balance and anti-aging. Polyphenols help encourage the growth of probiotics in your gut and in so doing fights growth of candida and yeast in your body. Flaxseeds are best used when ground in a coffee grinder to help in absorption in your digestive tract

Asian mushrooms

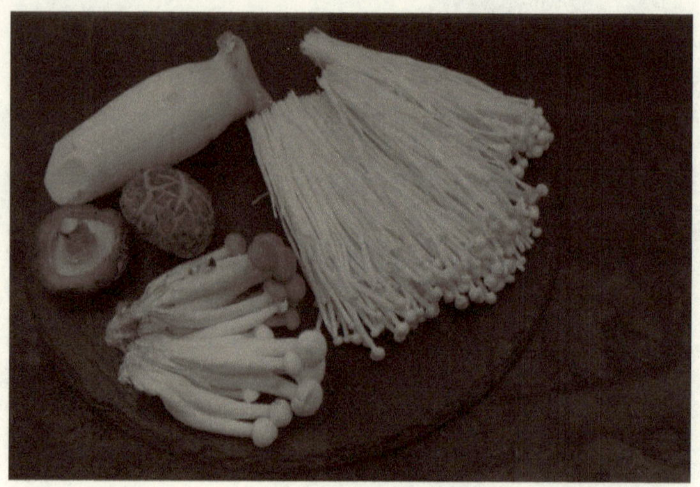

Mushrooms are beneficial foods, which help boost your immune system and ultimately fight inflammation. Some of the mushrooms you should take include lobster, oyster, Portobello, shiitake and maitake.

Berries

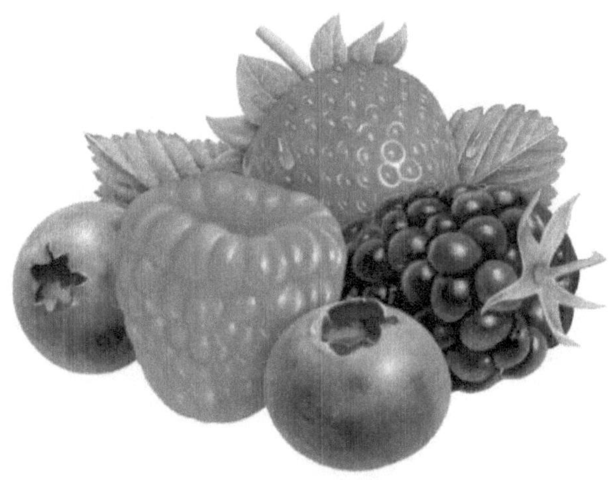

Berries are high in anti-oxidant properties (the tart cherries contain anthocyanin) that can help protect you from free radical damages. This can ultimately help protect your body from inflammatory responses. Some of the berries you should take include: blueberries, strawberries, blackberries, cherries, raspberries, cranberries and pomegranates. Taking a small quantity of berries can go a long way in minimizing damage to muscles. Anthocyanins help in restoring health and preventing further cell damage. That's why berries are very effective for intestinal inflammation and ulcerative colitis.

Papaya

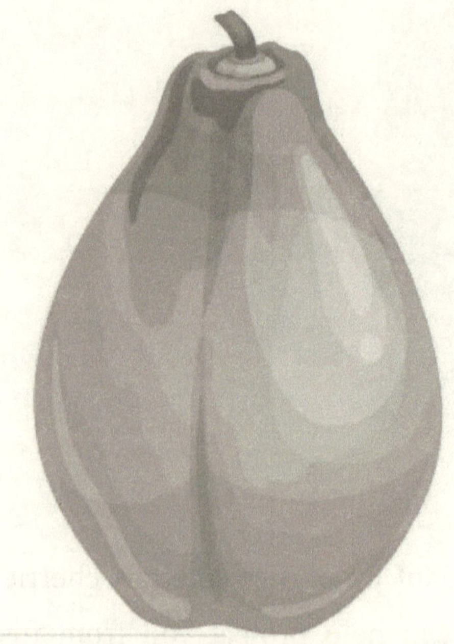

This fruit has an enzyme by the name of papin. This enzyme helps your body to reduce inflammation in the digestive tract. This means that taking papaya regularly can boost digestion greatly as well as fight any inflammation within the gut.

Beans

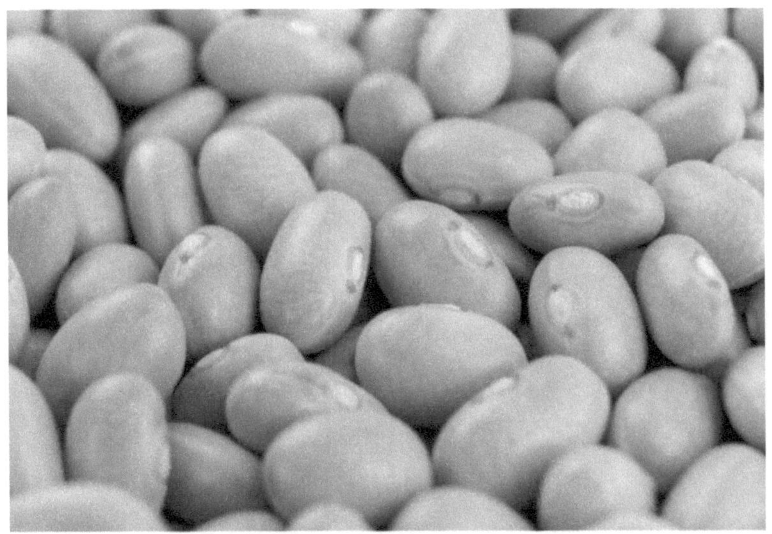

These are high in antioxidants, which are very effective for fighting inflammation. The good thing is that these are free from steroids, antibiotics and hormones, which are often found in animal-based proteins. Black beans are the best for fighting inflammation.

Olive oil

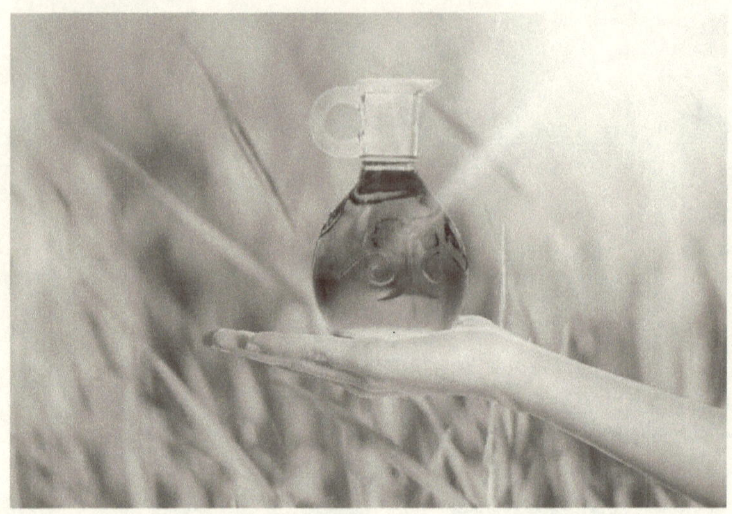

You should try extra virgin olive oil given that it is high in oleic acid and fatty acids, which have the ability to fight inflammation and pain. Use olive oil in sauces for a healthy snack.

Dark chocolate

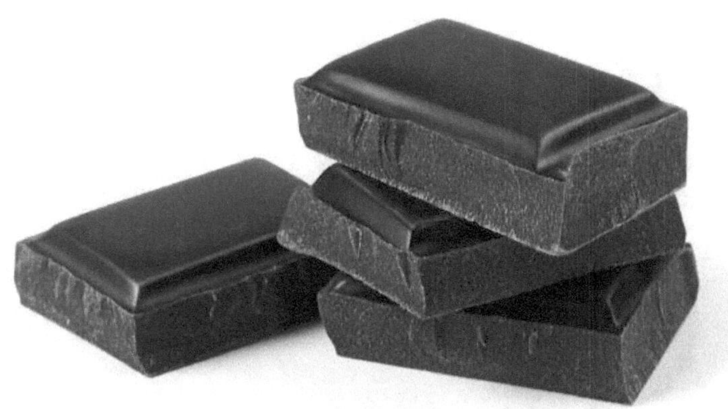

This has very great anti-inflammatory properties. As you take chocolate, ensure to avoid milk chocolate given that it is high in sugar and might not have the essential antioxidants that are in dark chocolate.

Pineapple

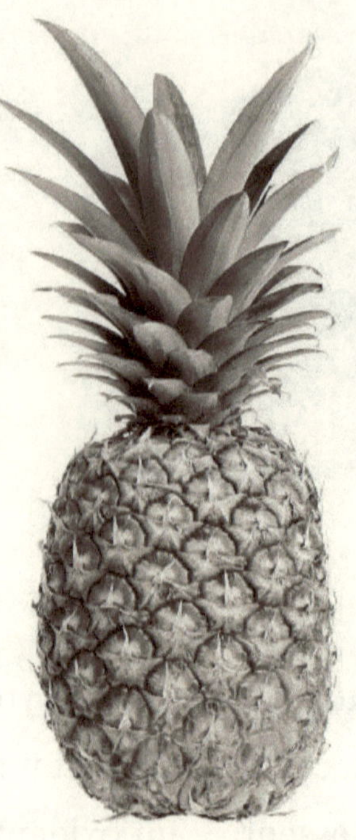

Pineapple has a compound called bromelain. This compound has the ability to reduce inflammation, reduce pain, bruises, and swelling, as well as digest food properly. This compound also helps prevent possible blood clot and also reduce risk of blood platelets building up on your blood vessels or sticking together. This greatly reduces occurrence of strokes or heart attacks and also boost heart health. Pineapple fruit also has high levels of vitamin C, potassium and vitamin B1 along with anti-oxidants that fight inflammatory diseases.

Apples

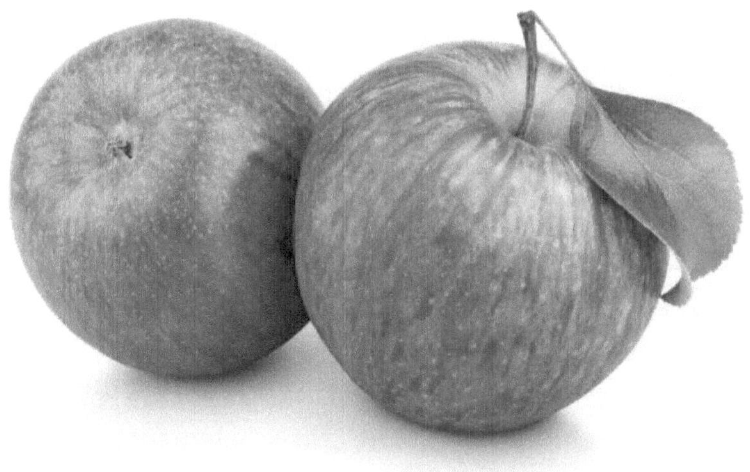

This nutritious fruit has a very important component in its skin and it goes by the name quercetin, a natural antihistamine, which works together with your body to deal with such threats like environmental allergies. It also helps in fighting inflammation in your body.

Spirulina

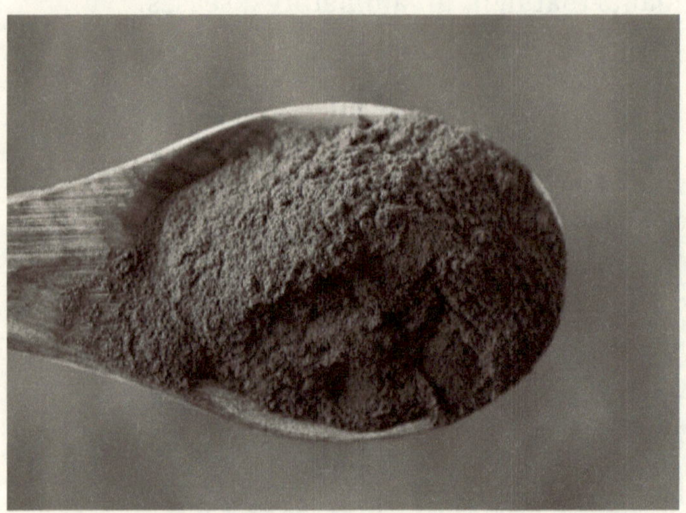

This algae has a blue-green color and is rich in amino acids, minerals and chlorophyll. The three elements normally combine to form an alliance of fighting and reducing inflammation.

Tea

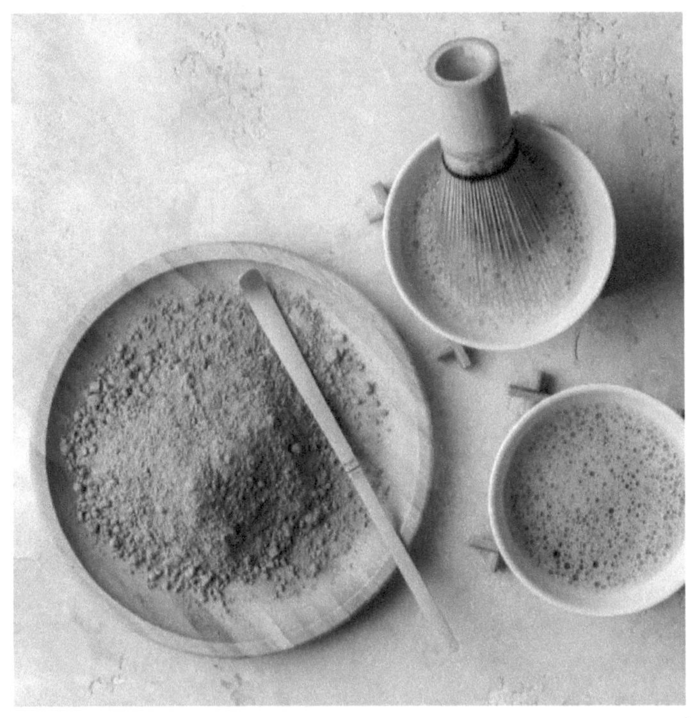

Matcha tea is the tea to go for if you want to get rid of inflammation. It has an impressive record of having an antioxidant, which is 17 times more powerful than the wild blueberries and 7 times stronger than dark chocolate. Its antioxidant properties help to fight inflammation in your body. You can purchase the best unfermented matcha powder from Japan where the best qualities come from. Tulsi is another beneficial tea, which is full of anti-inflammatory antioxidants and some other micronutrients, which maintain your heart health and your immune function.

Nuts

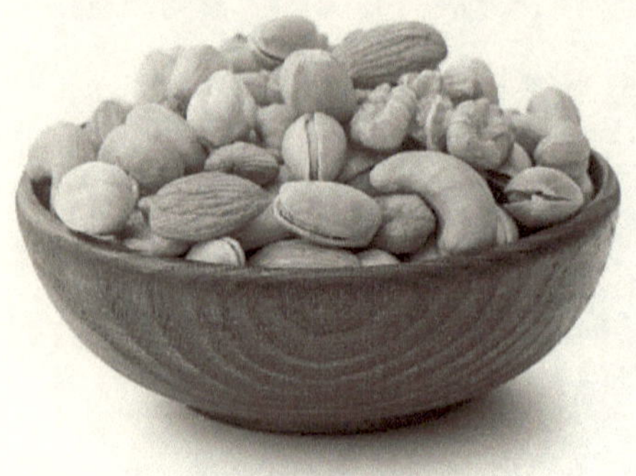

Different nuts are high in different fatty acids, vitamins and nutrients that help fight inflammation. For instance, walnuts are high in linolenic fatty acids while almonds contain high levels of vitamin E, calcium, fiber, and magnesium. There are also other nuts that are good at repairing damaged cells and fighting inflammation due to their antioxidant properties.

Whole grains

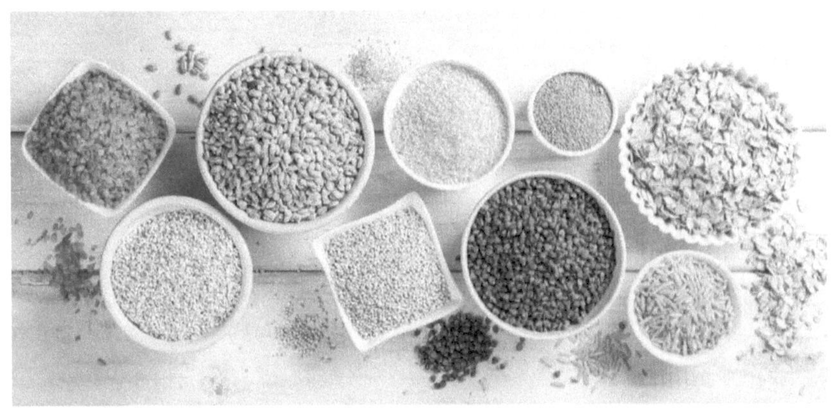

These are high in fiber, which is very effective for fighting C-reactive protein, which has been proven to cause inflammation. Some of the common sources of whole grains include oats, buckwheat, and brown rice. The whole grains help in stabilizing sugar and boost energy as well as fight inflammation.

Traditional food and fermented vegetables

As we have seen in the previous chapter, most inflammatory diseases start in the gut and this is as a result of imbalanced microbiome. Fermented foods and vegetables help to optimize your gut flora, which is good for a healthy immune system. In addition, it helps zone off chronic inflammation. Examples of some good quality fermented foods, which you incorporate in your diet, are miso, olives, natto, kefir, tempeh, sauerkraut, pickles, and kimchee. They all have the ability to re-fuel your gut with some beneficial bacteria. Fermented food also helps your body to get rid of harmful toxins like pesticides and heavy metals. The two are dangerous toxins that promote inflammation.

Bok Choy

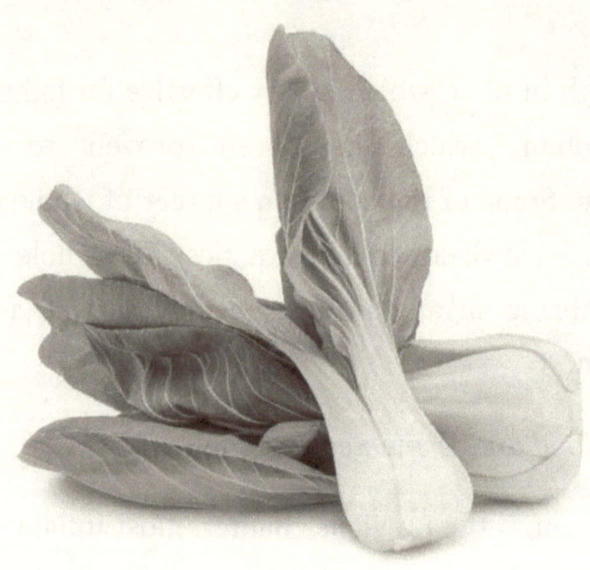

This Chinese cabbage has high amounts of minerals and at least 70 antioxidant ingredients among them hydroxycinnamic acids, important in fighting free radicals in the body. Bok choy can easily be incorporated in either

Chinese and global cuisines in various dishes to benefit from its anti-inflammatory powers.

Beets

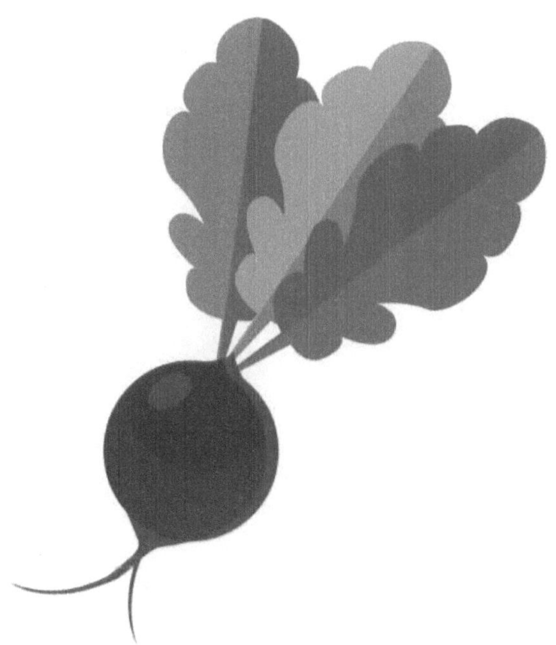

Known for their high levels of anti-oxidants, beets are very powerful in fighting anti-inflammatory agents in the body and aid in repair of cells and tissues damaged in the process. The most active ingredient in beets is referred to as *betalain* and is responsible for its deep red color and its anti-oxidant power. The vegetable also has minerals like magnesium and potassium, which helps a lot in repairing of damaged cells. In fact, deficiency of minerals such as magnesium is blamed for inflammatory reactions as the mineral is important in aiding detox. Magnesium deficiency inhibits utilization of calcium and this leads to buildup of calcium in tissues, a condition that is referred to as kidney stones. Such a situation is a kin to inflammation and can trigger other related complications.

Broth

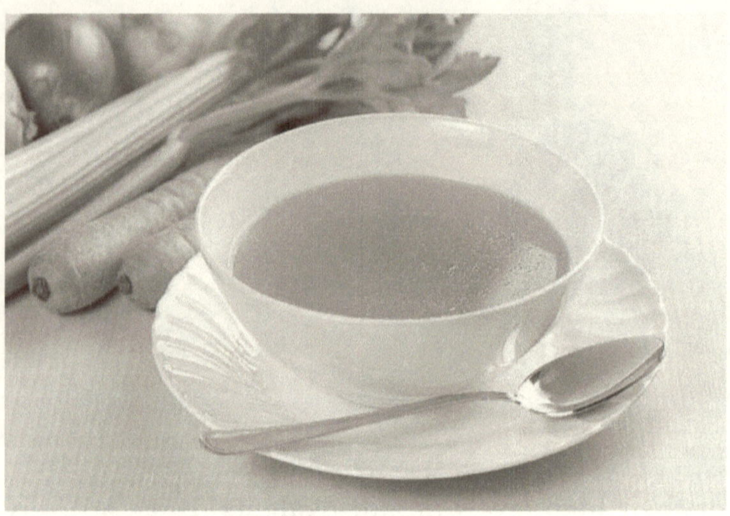

Bone broth has minerals such as phosphorus, magnesium, calcium and sulphur that the body can easily absorb. It also has glucosamine and chondroitin sulphates, two vital compounds usually sold in pharmaceutical supplements to fight joint pain, arthritis and general inflammation. Bone broth also contain amino acid, glycine and proline as well as collagen, substances that prevent gut inflammation and help in repairing damage cell walls especially if suffering from leaky gut syndrome.

Raw cacao

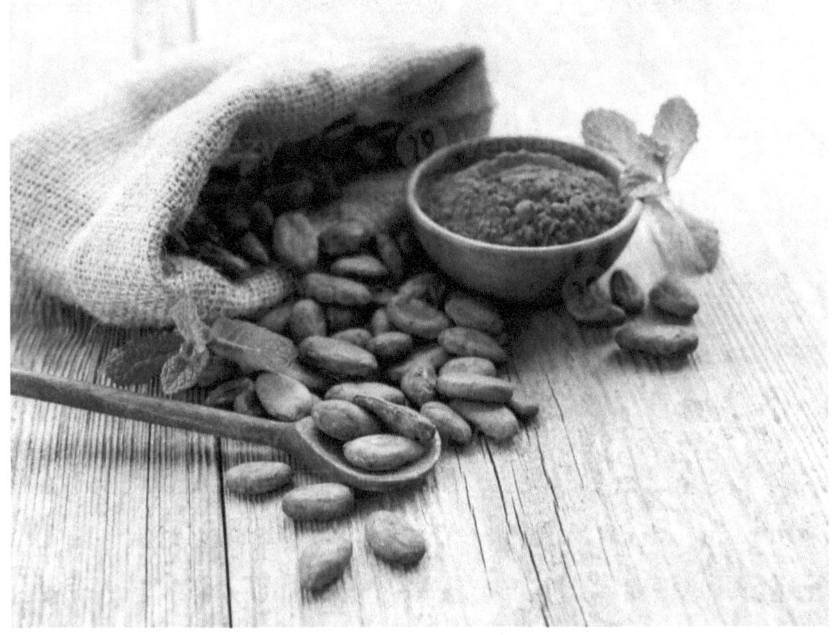

Cacao has at least 300 anti-inflammatory compounds, which makes it 20 times more powerful than blueberries in terms of its anti-oxidant power. When cacao is eaten raw, unprocessed and unsweetened, it has high amounts of minerals and antioxidant vitamins such as A and E. One way to enjoy raw cacao is to add it to smoothies or choose 70 percent cacao-rich organic dark chocolate to satisfy your sweet tooth.

Maca

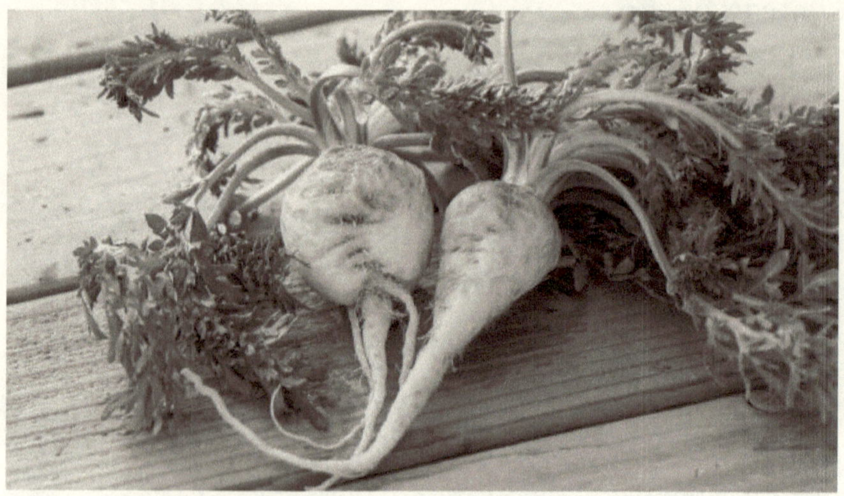

This is a South American based root that is usually used as a powder due to its potency and its ability to control bodily hormones. Maca also has high anti-oxidant power that makes it very powerful in fighting inflammation and repairing damaged cells.

Other fruits and foods for anti-inflammatory properties include

✓ Kiwi fruits

✓ Butternuts

✓ Okra

✓ Cloves

✓ Rosemary leaves

✓ Thyme

✓ Oranges

✓ Papirika

✓ Watermelon

2. Herbs & Spices That Fight Inflammation

It will surprise you to learn that herbs and spices have high antioxidant levels than even fruits and vegetables. They also contain other minerals and vitamins, which ensure that your meals have a huge amount of nutrient density. Studies have shown that herbs and spices have medicinal qualities so the next time you add them to your meals, you should know that you are upgrading your food. Let's look at some examples of herbs and spices you can use and how they can help your body.

Basil

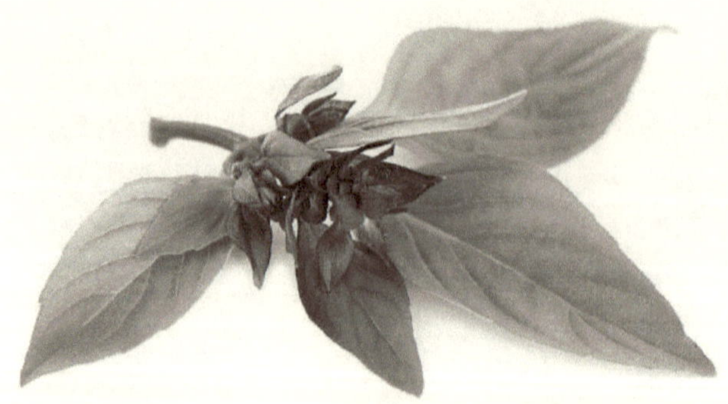

This herb is the perfect example of herbs that can fight inflammation. It contains a substance called Eugenol, which is responsible for providing basil with its smell and taste but most importantly, it has properties that can reduce inflammation.

Ginger

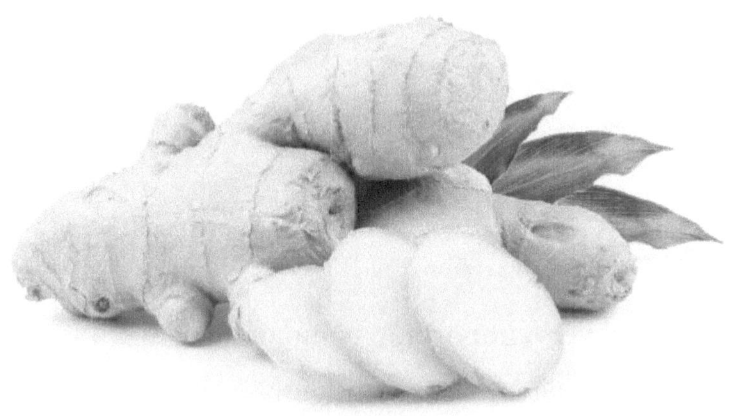

Ginger is a popular herb, which is commonly found in most people's kitchen shelves. It is one of the powerful herbs with strong anti-inflammatory properties, which come from a combination of paradols, shogaols, gingerols and zingerone. You can kill two birds with one stone with ginger since it also has pain killing powers.

Turmeric

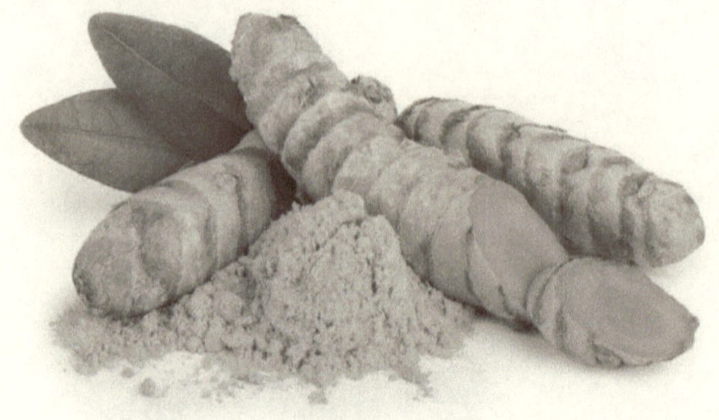

It contains a very important compound called Curcumin. This compound has numerous benefits including antioxidant properties that help protect the liver from the cellular damage, and properties that help control free radicals from damaging the cells. Cucumin also lowers the levels of histamine in your body resulting to reduced inflammation. Turmeric also contains iron, vitamin B6, and magnesium all of which give it anti-inflammatory powers. These 3 nutrients allow the red blood cells to grow and even maintain a perfect immune system. You can add turmeric to your smoothies, rice, soup etc.

Garlic

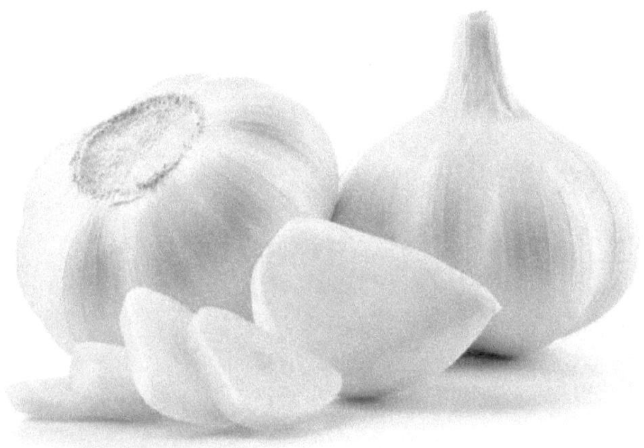

Garlic is very effective for fighting inflammation due to its high levels of sulfur compounds. When you take garlic, it is usually broken down to produce sulfenic acid, which has been proven to fight free radicals in your body. As you take garlic, it is important to moderate its intake in smoothies and in other foods. One way of ensuring that you take sufficient amounts of garlic is through roasting, or spreading on crackers. You can even crush it before incorporating in other dishes.

Cayenne

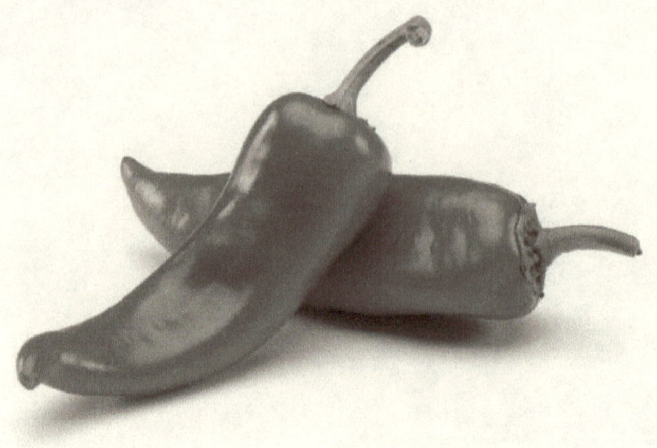

Cayenne and most hot peppers consist of a compound called capsaisin. This compound is used to block COX-2, which is an enzyme that takes part in inflammation processes that give birth to arthritis and a couple of other inflammatory diseases. It also has a minor advantage that come from its excessive heat when ingested. The amount of heat you get from it can help reduce the heat caused by inflammation in your body.

Oregano

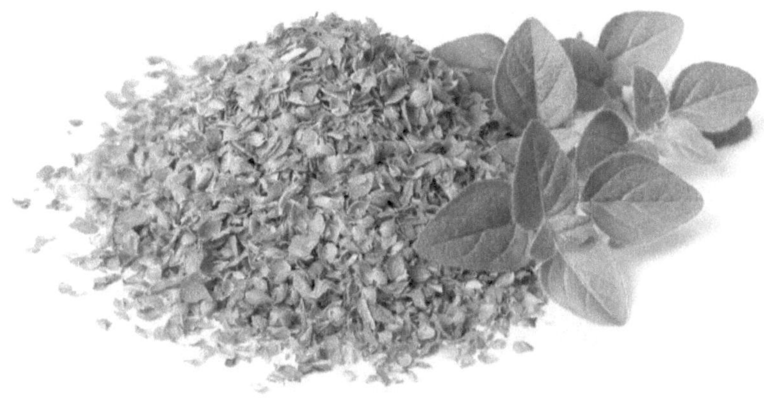

Oregano is good in fighting free radical production in the body and also helps with the damaged done in your body. It has two super components, which are bioflayanoids and polyphenols. These two are the compounds responsible for the reduction of inflammation.

White willow bark

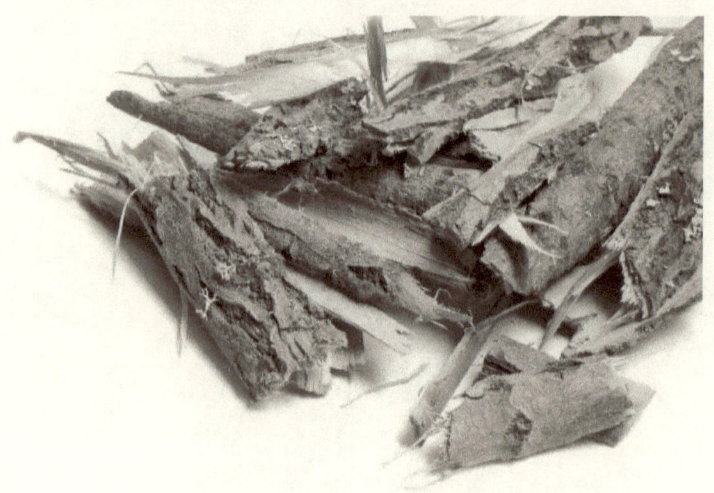

It is a very unique bark, which consists of a compound called salicin. This compound is similar to acetylsalicylic acid (Aspirin) the only difference being that it lasts longer than Aspirin. Salicin is a good pain reliever and has strong anti-inflammatory effects.

As you have probably seen, the best dietary plan for preventing or treating existing inflammation is through a healthy and balanced diet; primarily a plant based balanced diet. This means that a lot of fruits, vegetables, fiber and a lot of sea food protein are highly recommended. But for such a diet to work for you, there's need to avoid foods high in sugar and caffeine as these may serve to worsen inflammatory responses. And sadly, this will make all gains you have made useless. The only way to prevent that from happening is by avoid the "bad guys" as far as inflammation is concerned.

Let's get to that next.

Avoid Foods That Trigger Inflammation

Even though there is no single diet that you may be recommended to take as someone suffering from inflammation, it's a plain fact that some foods only serve to aggravate your symptoms. For that reason, you should stay away from foods that cause inflammation some of which include the following:

1. Unhealthy fats

The key culprit here is trans fatty acids commonly referred to as trans fats and most of saturated fats particularly from vegetable oils. According to research, unhealthy or processed fats are risk factors for inflammatory-related diseases such as diabetes, obesity and heart disease. Foods high in saturated fats are also likely to have high amounts of inflammatory omega 6 fatty acids, which without proper balance with omega 3 fatty acids are dangerous for you. Sad though, reports show that our diet has between 14 to 25 times of disease-promoting omega 6 fatty acids compared to healthier omega 3 acids!

2. Dairy

Dairy products such as milk, butter, cheese and yoghurt are very high in inflammatory sugars and proteins. Among these products is lactose, a type of sugar that majority of our metabolism cannot properly digest. Dairy products also have another protein called casein, that its digestion in the body produces inflammatory substances.

Funny enough, it happens that some arthritis patients who are milk intolerant have antibodies that help protect the body against the perceived threats. While this sounds alright, be aware that such antibodies may attack other parts of the body in what is called auto immune responses leading to chronic inflammation. For this reason, you are advised to reduce dairy intake and instead try its alternatives such as soy, almond or rice milk.

3. Meat

It is important to note that even though the terminology "meat" refers to animal meat in general, some meats such as fish are very beneficial in combating inflammation. Meats that should be avoided are meats high in cholesterol, most particularly the red meat. In fact, switching to a vegetarian diet can help reduce inflammation side effects as the diet bans eating meat, which is generally associated with high fat, calories and a general unhealthy lifestyle. In addition, the fats in such types of meat are often metabolized into inflammatory chemicals in the body.

Be aware that meats that are not marketed as organic but rather as vegetarian-fed or corn fed are pro-inflammatory. Such meats have high amounts of inflammatory chemical called *arachidonic acid* that, once it gets into body cells, triggers what is referred to as "the PGE2 pathway". Forget the fancy name here; any processes linked to arachidonic acid are simply inflammatory and you should be warned beforehand about the same.

4. Sugary treats and refined sugar

Even though some carbohydrates are essential to our dietary needs, refined sugars and sweets are not. Some sugars such as high fructose corn syrup are "poison" to the body, particularly if you have high blood sugar or other metabolic diseases. Failure of the body or its hormones to break down and fully metabolize refined sugar leads to damage of various cells or other complications such as high blood pressure.

As you should know by now, studies have already shown that limiting refined grains, avoiding simple carbohydrates and eating less processed sugars is a key factor in fighting inflammation. You need to replace those refined carbs with whole grains as these are a complete source of nutrients your body needs to fight inflammation. Consider buying whole grains in the form of fermented sourdough as fermentation let nutrients to be broken into simple units easily utilized in your body.

5. Some fruits and veggies

Apart from processed foods such as cured meats, candy bars and those with corn syrup, did you know that some fruits and veggies can be a disaster when it comes to inflammation? Actually, nightshade veggies among them eggplants tomatoes and potatoes have an ingredient called solanine, a substance that can worsen body pains and cause inflammation too. Furthermore, you could be sensitive to citrus fruits among them oranges along with tropical fruits such as pineapples, mangos and papayas. For this reason, you may need to reduce intake of these foods particularly if your inflammatory-related symptoms do not seem to improve.

Apart from specific foods, there are other ingredients or natural substances that can help prevent and treat inflammation ranging from supplements to essential oils. Let's discuss a few of these organic remedies:

Other Natural Remedies for Inflammation

1. Supplements: Anti-Inflammatory Natural Supplements

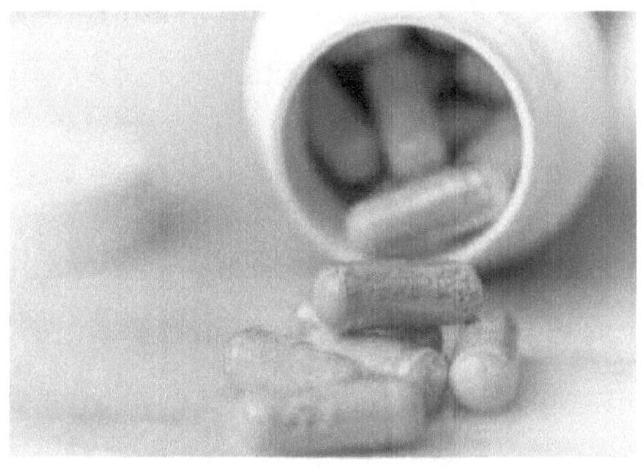

- Add quality multivitamin in your diet

You should supplement your diet with vitamins in order to increase nutrients in your body. Below are some examples of vitamins you should add and how they can help you to fight inflammation.

Vitamin D has anti-inflammatory effects. Examples of foods rich in vitamin D are eggs, mushrooms, and fish oils.

Vitamin C and B are very good when it comes to getting rid of free radicals that promote inflammation. To get vitamin C, you can take spinach, broccoli and lemons while for vitamin B, you can take potatoes, bananas, and nuts.

Vitamin E helps your body to reduce the level of CRP in the blood. You can get this type of vitamin by taking in sunflower oil, avocado, tomato, and whole grain products.

Other beneficial supplements

There are other supplements, which can help you fight inflammation naturally. Some of them include sulfur, glucosamine and chondroitin. The main goal of these supplements is to delay the development of the increased symptoms of joint inflammation.

2. Cannabis oil (CBD oil)

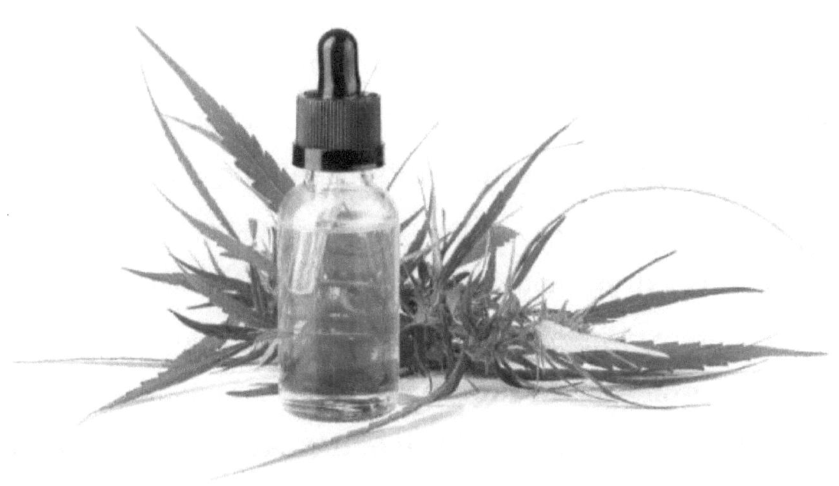

This is one of the most vital ingredients in the cannabis, or marijuana, a flowering herb that has palmate compound leaves and 5 to 7 saw-like or serrated leaflets.

Cannabis has more than 60 active compounds called cannabinoids, which trigger the cannabinoid receptors that occurs naturally in the body. One of these "cannabinoids" is cannabis oil, which has active ingredients that can help suppress pain related with inflammation such as the tetra-hydro-cannabinol (CBD). Cannabinol works by activating the same brain areas as the opioids thus can produce an analgesic effect. Your endocannabinoid system is tasked with monitoring the synaptic transmission in pain pathways. This means that these active ingredients act as neuro-modulators for various physiological processes such as sensation to pain.

Since cannabis oil has anti-inflammatory powers, it can help combat conditions such as arthritis, cancer among others. For instance, patients suffering from fibromyalgia normally depend on various opioid pain medications, anti-inflammatory drugs and corticosteroids. But a 2011 research that was done to investigate the suitability of cannabis oil in treating fibromyalgia showed promising results. The study had used 56 participants and half of these relied on medicinal marijuana, and it's this particular group that saw a great reduction on fibromyalgia symptoms and pain. The control group that used other traditional methods didn't note any traceable improvements on their inflammatory condition.

In addition, a study by Sean McAllister, a scientist, shows that cannabis oil can indeed hinder proliferation of cancer, its metastasis alongside growth of tumor. To be more specific, his study on *breast cancer* revealed that high dosage of CBD from cannabis oil lead to suppressed number of cancer cells. This undoubtedly shows that the active ingredient in cannabis oil can act as an inhibitor for cancer-causing gene, and cancer patients can benefit from this non-toxic therapy.

Furthermore, CBD can treat other inflammatory conditions among them bowel disorders, nausea, diabetes and auto-immune disorders. Like in Brazil, a 200mg of CBD daily administered to anticonvulsant epilepsy patients worked for 6 out of 7 patients to either reduce seizure or heal seizures completely. A dose of CBD can lower chances of heart attack by about 66 percent, and can also help prevent and control diabetic condition. A study done by a researcher called Mechoulam on mice suffering from type I diabetes showed good results. Since diabetes usually manifests around 14 weeks, mice were administered with CBD for the first 7 weeks after birth and later after another 7 weeks. From his findings, only 30 percent of the mice developed diabetes as compared to those administered with placebo.

Right from joint pain to the awkward irritable bowel syndrome, cannabidiol has shown to regulate both the acute and chronic inflammatory conditions through a couple of mechanisms. To some extent, the effect of CBD is even stronger than well-known foods like curcumin, antioxidants like veggies and resveratrol and vitamin C from fruits. For instance, the cytokines are proteins that are both secreted and synthesized by your immune cells once they've been stimulated. These are modulating factors that help balance the level of inflammation and how fast one can recover from such effect.

When it comes to fighting pain and inflammation, CBD and hemp oil work directly on what is referred to as cytokines. These are a broad category of small proteins produced by immune cells such as mast cells, B lymphocytes and macrophages. In other words, cytokines are modulating factors that help balance the level of inflammation and how fast you can recover from chronic inflammation.

So what's the link between CBD oil and the cytokines?

First, the cannabidiol in cannabis oil works by stopping the excess production of cytokine by immune cells and by reducing the production of cytokines by the T-helper cells. T-cells such as Th1 and Th2 are the similar cells where their over activity may trigger autoimmune responses and common food intolerances. CBD also helps reduce the level of interleukin-6 (IL-6), an inflammatory compound. On one scientific study, the effect of CBD was tested on 4 cell mediating molecules that are linked with inflammation to the intestines as well as the oxidation damage occurring at the gut.

The findings show that cannabidiol helps reduce the over-expression of Inducible nitric oxide synthase, a condition that leads to high-output of production nitric oxide (NO). The excess amount of NO is linked to the oxidation damage to your intestines through the reactive oxygen species abbreviated to as ROS. In addition, CBD and hemp oil has been found to help lower Interleukin-1β – levels, thereby reducing occurrences of inflammation that may lead to intestinal injury. IL-1β is reported to amplify the synthesis of immune system cells called leukocytes, a process that results into an inflammatory response.

This research proved that CBD actually inhibits release of inflammatory substances, which in a big way help restore your intestinal health. The reduction of reactive oxygen species and Inducible nitric oxide synthase by cannabidiol demonstrates the vital therapeutic roles of the CBD and hemp oil in reduction of colonic inflammation by indirect reduction of oxidative damage. CBD also helps restore interleukins IL-1B and IL-10 to normal behavior in order to lower chances for colonic inflammation setting in. In so doing, CBD can help treat related conditions such as bloating, gas, gut inflammation and constipation.

Nowadays, many NFL athletes have adopted CBD from cannabis extracts in a bid to manage symptoms of post head injuries and to control the chronic aches and pains after gaming. CBD can help athletes and other people working out to reduce inflammation levels while curbing stress and anxiety; without worry of testing positive for THC, which is banned by Athlete's Federation. So whether the chronic or casual pain you're facing is caused by inflammation or other related causes, CBD oil can help a lot.

Before we learn how you can effectively self-administer CBD rich oil, you should get to learn the most commonly available CBD products that you can choose from. Such products should come in handy when you need to get that remedy from stress, inflammation, pain and other related condition.

Here is what you should consider:

1. Hemp Oil

You should be aware that apart from cannabis or marijuana plant, CBD is also found in another plant referred to as **hemp**. Also referred to as "the industrial hemp", this is a high growing tree variety of cannabis genus that is grown for its suitability in production of fiber, seeds and oil. Then hemp oil is an ingestible product in liquid form that is made from various hemp plant materials or extracts through chemical processes. To use hemp oil, you can mix the CBD oil from hemp to smoothies or soups or take the already prepared capsules.

2. High CBD Cannabis Strains

This option is only possible if you're living in a marijuana approved state where sale or administering of high-CBD strains is legal. Such breeds often contain the psychoactive THC compounds in trace quantities thus shouldn't trigger any high effect even at higher dosage. You can choose between various marijuana or cannabis based extracts such as tinctures and topical.

3. Cannabis Tinctures

These are basically cannabis extracts that are obtained when soaked in either vegetable glycerin or alcohol and are applied under your tongue. Compared to other extracts, tinctures are easily absorbed into the body and can allow immediate change of dosage. Furthermore, the method yields a concentrated medicinal extract that can be preserved for long periods. This is because a tincture will maintain the medicinal value in a stable and soluble form as no volatile ingredients may escape in a case of heat processing.

To make a tincture, you have to obtain the concentrated form of the hemp extract or plant materials using ethanol as your solvent. Alcohol is the most preferred solvent though you can choose apple cider vinegar or vegetable glycerin. To start with, chop the plant materials, and then grind the roots or dry the leaves to obtain the primary extract. Then dissolve the extracts in the chosen solvent and stir until it fully dissolves. The resulting soluble extract will be same as the alcohol-prepared tincture though it might not be as concentrated.

Tinctures from cannabis were some of the earliest forms of medicines before they were banned in US. Since tinctures are less concentrated compared to other CBD oil extracts, they can be good remedies for stress relief or other mild symptoms. However, for strong and chronic ailments, other forms of CBD oil should be a better alternative.

4. Cannabis Topicals

These infused drugs are popular for aches and pains, and are generally applied directly onto the skin. Topicals usually offer localized relief and has other therapeutic compounds apart from CBD. In case you need to treat mild conditions back at your place of work, consider carrying salves and balms as they're non-psychoactive.

Nowadays, medical experts are coming up with recommended dosage for various CBD products like medicinal hemp and its oil, medical marijuana as well as other approved cannabidiol extracts. For instance, CBD rich hemp oil can come in various forms or concentrations say as capsules, thick paste or salves etc. You can also opt for CBD vapor, edible CBD-rich gum or candies that contain the same compounds in CBD oil. At first, your aim should be to start small and then increase your dosage gradually until you achieve the intended feeling.

With that in mind, let's see how you can use CBD and hemp oil for various inflammatory related conditions:

How to Use CBD and Hemp Oil

The main method of taking any of the two CBD extracts is orally, where you eat a concentrated paste or use tincture of drops. To take CBD in form of oil, try to hold it under your tongue in order for it to be absorbed in the mouth before you swallow. It's vital to do so since some of the CBD might be broken by your digestive system and hence may not get absorbed to various organs.

Another variation to take the drug orally includes mouth strips, capsules and other edible foods like chocolate bars. A starting point for CBD and hemp oil should be around 25mg of CBD administered twice daily. Then you should increase the dosage of CBD by 25 mg every 3-4 weeks until you get sufficient relief.

Another alternative to sublingual use is to obtain hemp in form of E-liquid also referred to as vape oil. The application of the vape oil depends on the product you buy though you'll likely need a vaporizer for this. Using the oil through a vaporizer is a powerful way to take the CDB oil as it easily and quickly get into the system. In what is referred to as "vamping", the oil enters the bloodstream through the lungs and so can quickly help you relax and fight stress-related inflammation. You can also purchase a vape kit that comes with a disposable vape cartridge which screws into the vaporizer. Having a disposable vape cartridge is important as it curtails the need to maintain the vaporizer pen. If you are to have a re-usable pen, you'll need to replace the coil or tank now and again.

But in case your symptoms begin to worsen; you should reduce the intake of cannabis oil to optimal 25 mg per day. You bear in mind that the concentration of the CBD oil in extracts depends on the method of preparation! Some extracts can have 1 mg per dose and other hundreds of milligrams; which should enable you to get any dosage in whatever form you prefer.

3. Essential Oils

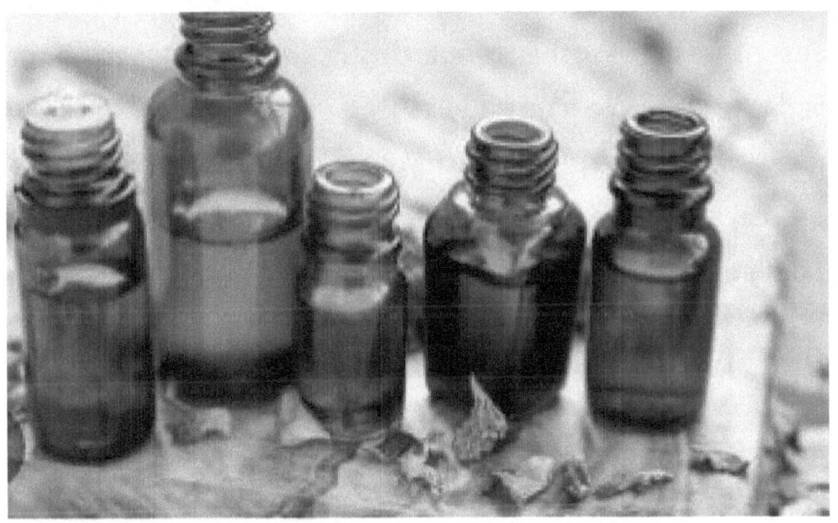

Essential oils are basically the fragrant, highly concentrated natural compounds that come from various parts of plants such as flowers, roots, bark, stems and seeds. These oils are also known as volatile oils or ethereal oils and are responsible for the distinctive smell in some plants. The oils are generally non-water based <u>phytochemicals</u> that are constituted of aromatic compounds. They are generally pure, crisp to the touch and are quickly absorbed by the skin; and that's they are widely applied through body massage.

Most essential oils range from clear to deep blue in color in their pure and unmodified form. Such natural oils from plants can help reduce either mild or chronic pains as well as related tension and inflammation that cause pain. Various pains can exist ranging from arthritis, joint pains, back pain, headaches, muscle pains and muscle spasms. While different medications could help relieve your pain, majority of them do pose negative side effects. Essential oils are natural and are also readily available; such as:

Lavender Essential Oil

Bathing in lavender oil is an effective way of fighting muscle and joint pain, and can help you sleep better stress-free, especially if you administer at bedtime. Lack of sleep may at times cause poor sleep so improving the amount and quality of sleep can help you monitor pain. For better results, you can blend equal amounts of chamomile and lavender to get improved sleep, reduced pain and stress-free experience. To do a lavender bath soak, obtain a bottle of pure lavender oil and add a few drops to your bath water.

Clary Sage oil

This essential oil can be added to various massage oils to relieve cramping, muscle spasms and muscle aches, in small amounts. The easiest way is to inhale clary sage in order to relieve tension in the nerves, lighten the mood and create a feeling of euphoria. However, ensure you don't use the oil with alcohol, as it can worsen the effects of drunkenness or cause complications.

Juniper essential oil

The oil has anti-spasmodic and anti-rheumatic abilities that allow it to reduce muscle pains, joint aches and muscle spasms. The most effective way is applying juniper as a cream or lotion, and has been used to treat chronic pains in arthritis and fibromyalgia. Juniper can also help strengthen the nerve and cease neuropathic pain, and may also act as a stimulant. Look for its cream or lotion form and apply before bedtime to sleep better.

Eucalyptus oil

This oil is mostly used topically on the skin due to its analgesic and anti-inflammatory properties. Eucalyptus oil is known to treat various problems that cause pain such as muscular aches and pain, strains, sprains and nerve pains. The oil can be used in cream or lotion form. Rub on the areas with pain, or use as salt in the bath or as a bath oil. To increase potency of the oil, you can add a few drops of lavender to diluted oil and carefully massage onto the painful areas. However, take caution since eucalyptus is toxic if used in high concentration or large amounts.

Rosemary oil

To treat arthritis-related problems like joint pains and muscle aches, rosemary can be of great help. The oil is also effective at boosting your memory, mental alertness and concentration, where it can still offer antidepressant effect. You can easily blend rosemary with other oils such as lavender, chamomile, peppermint and clary sage.

Peppermint Oil

If you suffer from painful inflammatory side effects, you can benefit from the healing power of peppermint. To treat the pains, just blend 4 drops of peppermint with a tablespoon of carrier oil like olive, coconut or jojoba. You can also add 2 drops of rosemary oil and a few drops of lavender to enhance potency and relieve strong pains. Apply carefully to the affected area ensure you keep away from the eyes. However, be aware that consuming the oil may trigger migraines and also worsen the pains if already affected.

Ginger oil

Ginger is known to improve mobility and ease back pain, and can help reduce muscle pains and sprains, rheumatic and arthritis pain. This oil is a powerhouse in its ability to reduce inflammation, relieve muscle pains and spasms and related pains. The oil can be blended with other essential oils such as rosemary and eucalyptus and then massaged on the skin topically. You can dilute or use undiluted amount of the oil to massage the skin to kill pain.

Yarrow oil

This one treats joint pains and aches as it is an anti-inflammatory oil and an analgesic pain reliever. To restore peace of mind and fight pain, dilute 4 drops of yarrow with 1-2 drops carrier oil and massage to the skin.

How to use oils for pain relief

Use 2-3 drops of essential oil and similar amount of carrier oil, such as jojoba, olive, coconut or olive oil. For oils like eucalyptus, you might need more amounts to avoid counteractive reactions on the skin. Use the oils around 2-4 times a day though you are free to adjust this depending on the intensity of the pain. To make oils more permeable to the skin, consider applying oil through a hot compress especially if dealing with severe or persistent pains.

Here are 3 ways in which you can use essential oil for pain relief:

1. Massage Technique

This is one the simplest methods you should adopt for a number of reasons. Topical application of essential oils triggers release of biochemical sensors that send signals that lower inflammation in cells. Based on studies, the body massage technique also helps cells to make new mitochondrial cells; a process that helps boost power-production centers within cells. A wide variety of essential oils such as lemon oil and lavender can be used directly on the skin in areas such as abdomen, tops and soles of feet, upper back, temples and the ears.

Use below guideline to treat various inflammation related pains through massage technique:

1. For joint pain and arthritis, massage few drops onto the area 1-2 times daily. In joint pains, try a hot or cold compress if your condition is intense. Chronic pains may require a hot compressor or a heating pad for duration of 30 minutes, 3 times daily.

2. Rub a few drops of diluted oil onto the affected areas 2-3 times daily or based on the intensity of the pain to relieve muscle pains. Muscle sprains should be massaged with diluted oil a number of times a day every 2-3 hours.

3. Bone spurs are best treated through a massage of 1-2 drops of oil for around 2-3 times daily. You should apply the oil consistently in order to facilitate a proper physical alignment.

Inhalation

Research has already proven that the aromatic properties of oils can heighten the senses and impact on your mind and body positively. This is because the scents produced by essential oils do stimulate the central nervous system, which controls feelings and emotions.

When you inhale a scented plant extract, the aroma is sent into your limbic system to boost the memory and your general feeling. This limbic system produces beneficial chemicals such as serotonin and endorphins that impacts on the central nervous system. Serotonin is useful in combating stress and anxiety; while endorphins are soothing to pain and can boost your sexual response. Through inhalation, oils can help relax your mood and diffuse into the respiratory and olfactory systems of the body.

There are many ways in which oils can be diffused in air, such as through steam, dry heat, mist or through a fan-assisted evaporation. An essential oil can also be inhaled directly from the bottle that came with it especially in circumstances that you do not have a diffuser. In addition, another simple and cost effective way to inhale the oils is to add a few drops into a bowl of water and then use a tea light candle to generate vapor.

Bathing with Essential Oils

This is a form of natural medicine where water at different temperatures is used to stimulate the various systems of your body. Reports show that winter swimming can help lower fatigue and tension while it boosts mood and relieve pain. If you suffer from painful conditions like rheumatism, asthma or fibromyalgia, water therapy with essential oils can help your general wellbeing. You don't have to do swimming to enjoy the benefits of hydrotherapy! You can simply add a few drops of the oil in bathing water, say about 10 drops, and then you allow the oils to be absorbed into the skin.

To bathe in essential oils, just add the specific oil before bathing but be aware that the volatile oil may evaporate if left in water for so long. If you find that bathing in oil wasteful, then consider applying the oil to your body a few minutes before bath to minimize any possible waste. You should however take extra care as specific scented oils may not be recommended to add to your bath. Essential oils such as lemon, clove, eucalyptus, aniseed, peppermint, spearmint and orange can sting your skin so for this reason only, use a few drops to avoid any counter reactivity or possible skin burns.

4. Avoiding Gluten Exposure

Gluten refers to proteins found in wheat's endosperm; which constitutes of 80% of all proteins found in wheat. The gluten protein nourishes the embryo of wheat seeds during germination that later affects the elasticity of dough when making baked products.

But why avoid gluten while it's the top ingredient in most baked foods? On top of being less nutritious, gluten protein in wheat, barley or rye isn't properly digested into amino acids like other proteins. This is because the protein breaks down in various *peptides* or short strings of amino acids, which can't be further broken down.

And if you suffer from celiac disease, each short chain of amino acid reacts in a manner that it increases the toxicity of other peptides. Celiac disease is a serious autoimmune response caused by gluten consumption, and is characterized by bloody or fatty stools, nausea, gas, diarrhea, stomach pain as well as appetite changes.

Worst still, sensitivity to gluten can lead to symptoms that correspond to celiac disease such as breathing problems, diarrhea, vomiting, facial swelling, hives and itchy rashes. Most of these symptoms occur because gluten causes *inflammation* in your small intestines especially if you are gluten intolerant or suffer from celiac disease.

But how can you know if you suffer from celiac disease or have any sensitivity to gluten for that matter? It's quite simple. In case you've never being tested for gluten sensitivity, you may decide to ditch wheat products for approximately 8 weeks and then gradually re-introduce wheat-based products. In case you felt better off without gluten foods and now you feel sick or experience various side effects, your woes could be linked to wheat allergies. Be aware that gluten sensitivity related to celiac disease along with other inflammatory responses may cause toxins and microbes to buildup in the blood stream leading to chronic inflammation.

Here, your entire body system gets overwhelmed, and it sends incorrect signals about what invaders to be destroyed. At the end, your immune system ends up destroying its own cells in what you already know is referred to as *autoimmune disease.*

Once sure that you're gluten sensitive or if at risk of celiac disease, these tips can help you reduce the amount of gluten in your diet:

1. Eat naturally gluten-free grains and cereals

Crackers, bread and pasta do contain gluten, but you don't have to ditch all cereals and grain to stay gluten-free. Grains such as tapioca, millet, corn, buckwheat, polenta, amaranth, teff and quinoa are naturally grain-free unless processed. Find a way to swap ordinary breadcrumbs using polenta crumbs, and use quinoa to make pasta and noodles. You can get gluten-free substitutes for foods like cereals, bread rolls, crackers, bread and pasta.

2. ***Try to eat plenty of protein-rich meat to replace iron-rich breads and cereals***. Some recommended meats that you can take are fish, but make sure that they are not covered with bread-batter. If you cannot tolerate these foods, consider eliminating them from your diet totally. Also, be aware that additives in bread-batter such as fillers, sugars and preservatives can affect your blood sugar and may also lead to some changes in your weight.

3. ***Make your own canned soups, sauces and stocks***. This is because majority of pasta sauces, condiments, stocks and gravies contains wheat flour and other gluten foods. Chicken stock and other canned soups contain a relatively high amount of gluten because they are thickened with

processed wheat flour. If in doubt, you can make your own pasta sauces or gravies using alternatives like potato starch, arrowroot starch and corn flour to thicken them. Also prepare your soup from scratch or choose gluten free varieties.

4. *Replace beer with wine or distilled spirits since it's made with malted barley that contains gluten*. Wines and distilled spirits are usually free from fruits and vegetables. In place of gluten-rich beers, ales, stouts and lagers, you can try out gluten-free alcohol such as liqueurs, spirits, sherry, wine and cider. These gluten-free beers are available in some local restaurants and supermarkets, but you should check the label to be sure.

5. Read food labels when you shop

Packaged foods should have a well-illustrated labeling that includes list of gluten cereals and other allergens used to make the product; regardless of how little gluten quantity is. In such labels, look for any mention of substances like wheat, spelt, oats, rye or Kamut; together with other grain that may have been breaded with gluten. In majority of brands or specific products, such ingredients could be highlighted in bold. If need be, adopt products from individual companies that sell gluten-free foods or instead order online especially if buying in bulk.

6. Stock your pantry well

In case you don't have sufficient time to make meals, you can prepare meals and keep them in the pantry or freezer. Ensure that you get gluten-free frozen meals from fish, breaded chicken, pasta or pizza. You'll find it easier to continue when you don't have to cook every time so take a break from the stove every once in a while.

7. Get a cookbook

Let's face it: deciding gluten-free foods for different meals could be such a nightmare. Here, you can choose to buy a gluten-free cookbook in order to get variety of recipes and fight 'boredom' that comes with specific meals. Look for books that have resources on gluten-free cooking and baking options from top sellers from Amazon and other sites. Also research online for ideas on possible substitutions you can make to ensure you don't compromise your gluten-free lifestyle. This book has <u>over 40 recipes</u> to help you get started.

8. Inquire how ready foods are prepared

When eating out, be aware that even naturally gluten-free foods are likely to be cross contaminated with gluten. For this reason, get to know details on how foods served in restaurants are prepared and the type of equipment used. As stated before, gluten-free foods are best made in separate utensils or pans and in pots that are thoroughly washed.

You already know that having persistent inflammatory and autoimmune reactions can trigger more dangerous ailments apart from heart diseases and diabetes, such as cancer and asthma. One of the most recommendable ways of fighting such related conditions is use of food as you have probably learnt. The best dieting lifestyle is through adapting a healthy diet comprising of less processed foods, no added sugars, low in fats and high in vegetables, fruits and whole grains. Such a diet is also of low-fat, nonfat dairy foods and of high omega 3 fatty acids.

Here are tips to help you choose various foods to both fight inflammation and to keep hunger pangs and cravings off:

Anti-inflammatory Diet Tips

To effectively use diet to address inflammation, ensure that you eat as much fresh foods as possible, comprising of abundant fruits and vegetables. Avoid taking processed or fast foods to prevent oxidative damage to the endothelial cells. The other consideration is the total number of calories you take daily, which largely depends on your age or activity. Your calorie intake should be based on these facts:

- An adult person normally needs about 2000-3000 calories daily

- Men and active people do need more calories as compared to women, children and less active people.

- Fluctuations of your body weight means that you aren't eating appropriate numbers of calories based on your level of activity.

- Calories distribution should be about 40-50 percent carbohydrates, 20-30 percent protein and 30 percent healthy fats.

- Ensure that your meals contain fat, proteins and carbohydrates

Carbohydrates

Based on a 2000 calories a day diet, as an adult man, you should consume about 240-300 grams of carbohydrates. If you are a woman, consuming between 160 to 200 grams is recommended. You must ensure that your carbohydrate diet plan does not include high concentration of sugar and wheat. These two ingredients are normally present in breads and other packaged snacks.

Protein

Your recommended daily calorie intake of proteins should be between 80-120 grams. However, you may need to decrease your protein intake especially if you have problems such as autoimmune disease, allergies or kidney problems. Beans are good sources of protein especially the soy beans. Reach for whole-soy foods that are available in various organic and unprocessed products.

Fat

Taking fat is recommendable in the ratio of 1:2:1, of polyunsaturated to monounsaturated to saturated fat. These fats are strictly recommended in that they directly fight inflammation. You need to minimize intake of saturated fats from vegetable based oils that are often digested into inflammatory products. Do so by taking little cream, high-fat cheese, butter, fatty meats, un-skinned chicken or products consisting of perm kernel oil.

For your main cooking oil, extra-virgin olive oil is recommendable. Organic canola oil that is expeller-pressed is good for a neutral tasting oil or a high-oleic, organic and expeller pressed safflower or sunflower oil. However, avoid mixed vegetable oils, cottonseed oil, corn oil, regular sunflower oils and safflower oil. Also avoid vegetable shortening or margarine, together with products that contain these oils as these fuel inflammation.

Fiber

You need about 40 grams of fiber, which you can obtain from whole grains, vegetables especially beans, and berries. If reaching for ready-made cereal, ensure you read the package to ensure they offer 5 grams of fiber for every ounce of serving.

Phytonutrients

These are nutrients required by your body in order to prevent age-related diseases from setting in. Such diseases include neurodegenerative disease, cancer and cardiovascular diseases. You need to eat variety of mushrooms, fruits and vegetables. Include cruciferous vegetables such as cabbages in the diet together with soy food.

Drinking tea instead of coffee is more beneficial, preferably if taking the good quality green, white or oolong tea. If you are a wine drinker, red wine is more advisable. To guide you on choosing the best food ideas for different meals, here is a recommended way to balance meals:

1. Breakfasts

The best approach for breakfast is to adopt natural ingredients found in your homemade smoothies from non-dairy yogurt, honey or berries. You can also go for those egg dishes, particularly those made from organic eggs to help lower inflammation. In case you want a toast, go for the gluten or wheat free toasts such as those from rice breads.

2. Snacks and appetizers

The most advisable type of snack is probably fresh veggies or a handful of fruits. Here, you can obtain a handful of snow peas or crispy apple. To add to the delicacy, you can chip in a handful of dates, an avocado, or stuff a big Portobello mushroom with kale or other greens. Nuts and fruits are important as snacks since they are filled with nutrients, fatty acids as well as minerals.

3. Soups and salads

For these, you require a healthy salad or soup that can impact on your inflammation. You should opt for miso soup containing gluten-free noodles or vegetable soup with a butternut squash base. Since you could be having an inflammatory response to nightshade fruits and vegetables, you may stay away from tomatoes or bell peppers soups. To make salads, you need fresh organic toppers with darker leafy greens such as broccoli. Remember that you can dress your favorite salad by sprinkling with olive oil or vinegar.

4. Main dishes

For a heavy but healthy meal, you need to go for fish, a rich source of omega 3 fatty acids. To get protein, chicken with tofu can really make a wonderful main dish. However, you should try as far as possible to avoid red meats, but instead go for organic or meat from grass-fed animals. Processed meats should not be considered as they contain harmful chemicals that may worsen your condition.

5. Desserts

You need to find a sweet dessert that doesn't compromise your goals to fight inflammation. In such a case, you can turn to a melted dark chocolate or some chopped fruits to obtain the antioxidants you require and vitamins. For creamy dessert, non-daily yogurt, vanilla extract or honey can make a good option. If your system is okay with milk, choose a non-fat or low-fat dairy such as a light ricotta cheese.

While following an anti-inflammatory diet is the right thing to do, it's a fact that doing away with your favorite foods such as wheat products, processed grains, refined sugar, red meat and processed dairy can be challenging at first. So if you find it hard to cut out these foods out of your diet all at once, try to gradually reduce the amount you consume until well adapted.

Moreover, it is important to understand that success in the diet all depends on being consistent *i.e.* only eating the recommended foods. To make this possible, the next chapter will have some helpful tips that will hold you by the hand on your journey to fighting inflammation.

Tips For Success: Success Tips In Starting And Staying On The Anti-Inflammatory Diet

When it comes to any new dieting lifestyle, the key to success is making consistent food choices. And when making such a lifestyle change, be aware that it isn't a life sentence but a choice. Another thing; you don't have to be hard on yourself or feel frustrated- take your time and make initial preparations. More precisely, it is advisable that you undertake the process step by step to make the transition effortless.

These tips can help you make it in the diet:

1. Be prepared for the transition

You don't have to relocate to anti-inflammatory regions or stress yourself into the diet as far you're prepared about it. For obvious reasons, it's not recommended that you transit directly into this strict diet; otherwise, you're likely to give up.

The initial step is to learn what to put on plate and those foods to avoid and then proceed to create a simple diet plan or come up with easy-to-prepare recipes. You can then stock your pantry with stuffs like hemp seeds, flax seeds, coconut oil and spices as these are long lasting and will perhaps be used in most recipes. If worried about the cost of ingredients, you should consider buying in bulk or at discounted prices from various food stores.

Basically, be ready to eat a lot of veggies, fresh fruits, legumes, sea foods and whole foods such as brown rice. For breakfasts, you don't have to cook daily but rather can go for smoothies made from fruits, veggies or healthy fats. For occasional snacks, look for unsweetened or unsalted nuts and seeds, and tofu as it's a good source of calcium and protein. With proper preparation, you can be ready to deal with common pitfalls and successfully adjust your lifestyle.

Note: Before you change to anti-inflammatory diet, consider talking to your doctor if you have any fears or health concerns regarding the new food choices.

2. Start Small

Begin with those simple meals that require locally available ingredients from supermarkets, groceries or local farmers markets. If you find it hard to switch to 100 percent anti-inflammatory diet foods, try to include a few anti-inflammatory ingredients in your everyday cooking for a start.

Get variety of foods by making a list of nuts and seeds, herbs or other ingredients to form part of your diet. For instance, start with fresh fruits for breakfast or fresh fruit smoothie each breakfast with some dairy.

Then try eating a salad for lunch and dinner, alongside beans, unsalted seeds, nuts and whole grains. Use fresh herbs and seasonings such as cinnamon, pepper, garlic, chilies, pepper, turmeric and other ingredients. Try adding hummus in various meals to boost flavor or eat it for snack, and add herbs in salads to complete the meal.

You also need to plan for possible substitutions for snacks or treats by having enough bites at coffee time or midnight. Ensure that you plan for your entire day's or week's supply of nuts, seeds and whole-wheat bites to avoid eating sugary or processed foods.

3. Limit Saturated Fat

While unsaturated fats can promote heart health and facilitate weight loss, avoid saturated fats as these build up LDL cholesterol and increase risk for heart disease.

In general, limit saturated fat that comes from red meat, cheese and butter. Do away with the saturated fat from red meat for healthy fats such as coconut or olive oil fish oil or oil from nuts. Instead, top your salads with nuts in place of cheese; use avocado for mayonnaise or olive oil in place of margarine. As stated before, unsaturated fatty acids like fish oil promote heart health by boosting HDL cholesterol.

HDL is the "good" cholesterol referred to as High Density Lipoprotein (HDL). This type of lipoprotein transports cholesterol away from your body and the liver, where it can then be excreted or recycled. However, the Lower Density Lipoprotein (LDL) carries the cholesterol from your liver to body tissues. Scientists are of the view that dieters with higher levels of HDL are less likely to develop cardiovascular problems like the heart disease. The simplest way to boost the level of HDL is to eat lots of healthy fats, as this reduces your triglycerides to HDL ratio. As opposed to saturated fats like hardened vegetable oils, most healthy fats are liquid in room temperature.

4. Choose Satiating Foods

Majority of wheat based snacks and junk foods contain substances linked to weight gain, obesity, heart disease, diabetes and related health problems. So aim to eat foods rich in fiber such as veggies, oat bran, dried beans, flaxseeds and fruits such as citrus, apples and strawberries.

Dietary fiber is recommended, as it doesn't raise your blood sugar level, as it slows down glucose absorption into the blood. Fiber also assists in production and storing of fats in the body, besides making you feel fuller for longer and fighting cravings. Low glycemic and fiber-rich veggies like artichokes, asparagus, summer squash and broccoli should be top on your priority foods, as will keep you satiated.

Some of the best sources of fiber are fresh fruits, their seeds and pulp, the soft, wet and fleshy part of the fruit. Focus on fiber-rich and low-glycemic fruits among them bananas, oranges, pears, peaches, water melon, grape fruit, green apples and berries. Also add legumes to your diet such as kidney beans, pinto beans, white or black beans, lima beans, soybeans and chick peas.

5. Eat More Vegetables

These plant based foods are nutrient-packed and thus helps you boost your nutrients intake and keep you healthier. Veggies help shrink the belly fat and aid in total body fat loss, due to their ability to satiate you and help you reduce calorie intake.

They are also low in carbs; thus, you can eat high amount without altering blood sugar levels or gaining body fat. According to research, a huge proportion of belly fat is reduced when you fight inflammation. Eating a meal full of vegetables provides you with all the vitamins, fiber and minerals that you need to support healthy metabolism and keep off inflammatory reactions.

6. Only Eat Fresh Fruits

There are various reasons to choose fresh fruits, ranging from being sweet and nutritious to being rich in minerals such as potassium and vitamins. Potassium is good at controlling blood pressure while vitamins such as A and C helps promote a healthier immune system.

And while fresh fruits are recommended, this is not the case with fruit juices or processed fruit concentrate. Unknown to make dieters, these have higher calorie level and can hinder effective weight loss. When choosing fruits, go for those unprocessed variety; though canned, frozen or dried fruits with no added ingredients or sweeteners are acceptable. Also limit intake of fruit to below 2 cups a day to reduce intake of carb or fructose that may affect weight.

7. Take More Whole Grains

Research has shown that whole grain can aid weight loss and reduce Basal Metabolic Index compared to processed grains. Whole grains are important for facilitating lesser belly fat and lower body mass indexes for a number of reasons. They are lower in fat, contain no cholesterol and have high amounts of antioxidants, fiber, vitamins and minerals. Eating unprocessed grains can help you balance blood sugar, reduce calorie intake due to high fiber content and feel fuller for longer, facilitating weight loss.

Whole grains also contain higher nutritional content than processed grains which vital parts such as bran and germ has been removed. To accelerate weight loss and boost health, choose whole grains from foods such as whole wheat products, quinoa, oats and brown rice. If you've been eating processed grains such as white floor and rice, replace white rice with the brown variety and processed oats with the rolled oats. The key is to avoid the packaged refined carbs such as cakes, crackers and cookies, as these are junk food with added sugars.

8. Only eat necessary carbs

While eating variety of whole-grain foods made with complete grain kernel is important, you may need to eat such foods in moderation if seeking to reduce carb intake. Knowing the quantity of carbs you take can help you determine calorie intake especially if seeking to lose weight. Ideally, you should eat small quantities of non-starchy kind of carbs to help limit number of calories preferably from complex carbohydrates like grain breads and legumes. Additionally, you should incorporate more veggies in your diet. Get rid of the high carb foods and snacks in your fridge and replace with such stuff like lean meat, shell fish, fresh fish and low carb gluten-free snack bars. Also learn to read food labels especially for packaged foodstuffs.

9. Choose snacks wisely

Snacking on a handful of nuts has shown to facilitate fat loss in a more effective way than other food stuffs like ice cream, chocolate or wheat based products. Nuts such as almonds helps you remain full and fight occasional hunger, while keeping your metabolism revved up. Both nuts and seeds are high in fiber and proteins, which make them a snack you can't resist. Apart from fiber and protein, nuts and seeds have mono and polyunsaturated fatty acids, which can reduce cholesterol level and improve heart health. They have high amounts of omega 3 fatty acids which help eliminate cholesterol, cure heart problems, cure inflammation and improve the nervous system.

You can try eating Asian snacks among them dried anchovies and kelp chips prepared in coconut or palm oil. You can also fry your own snacks, by simply frying them using non-inflammatory oils such as olive or coconut oil. To increase your snack options, fry veggies such as peppers and onions in lard or coconut oil until crisp. You should eat at least 2 gluten-free snacks per day especially after breakfast, after lunch and dinner. Doing so helps you remain full for longer, and makes it possible to keep off wheat based and processed snacks.

10. Eat mineral-rich foods

You should know that lack of essential minerals or electrolytes in your body can lead to low blood pressure, mineral imbalances and sluggishness. The symptoms to loss of electrolytes may be interpreted as low blood sugar and can make you discontinue the diet.

The rule of the thumb here is to consume about 300mg of magnesium and 100grams of potassium daily. Magnesium is a co-factor in more than 300 enzymes in your body, and helps regulate various biochemical functions in your body. The mineral is also required by the body to synthesize the DNA and monitor the heartbeat. One way to boost the level of magnesium in the body is to eat an ounce of cashew-nuts or roasted almonds for your snacks.

11. Boost intake of antioxidants

Antioxidants are simply chemicals that destroy free radicals in the body, and work by inhibiting oxidation in the cells. When oxidation occurs, it can cause damage to the cells by setting in motion a chain reaction from the production of free radicals in the cells. As this chain reaction can cause damage, and/or death to the cells, antioxidants act to prevent this through elimination of the chain reaction. Your body produces antioxidants on its own, known as endogenous antioxidants, to neutralize free radicals. However, the level of these antioxidants is not enough, and you therefore need to upgrade the concentration from external sources, primarily the diet, otherwise known as exogenous antioxidants.

A diet high in antioxidant is a proven cure for most inflammatory reactions particularly if high in fruits and veggies. These two ingredient categories are super foods when it comes to fighting inflammation, as they contains less fat, high fiber content and cancer-fighting minerals. In fact, a diet high in fruits and veggies can lower risks associated with bladder, breast, pancreases and larynx cancers. They also have high quantities of antioxidants like selenium, vitamin C and E as well as beta-carotene.

As far as fruits and veggies are concerned, you can get anti-oxidants from specific antioxidant groups such as:

- Vitamin A – sources include food like sweet potatoes, milk, liver, carrots, and egg yolks

- Vitamin E – comes from vegetable oils (e.g. wheat germ oil), nuts, whole grains avocados, and seeds

- Beta-carotene – from fruits and veggies like mangoes, carrots, parsley pumpkin, apricots, and spinach

- Lycopene –commonly available in tomatoes as well as other foods like pink grapefruit and watermelon

- Polyphenols –oregano and thyme

- Anthocyanins – these include fruits and veggies among them grapes, eggplant and berries. These antioxidants can fight a number a cancers such as brain and blood cancers.

- Flavonoids – green tea, red wine, apple tea, citrus fruits, and onion

- Isoflavonoids – tofu, peas, soybeans, lentils, and milk

- Lutein – green and leafy vegetables like spinach and corn

- Manganese – lean meat, nuts, seafood and milk

- Selenium – offal, whole grains seafood, and lean meat

- Vitamin C – blackcurrants, mangoes, spinach, strawberries, oranges, kiwifruit, broccoli, and capsicum

- Allium sulphur compounds – onions leeks, and garlic

- Cryptoxanthins –pumpkin, mangoes and red capsicum

- Indoles – cruciferous vegetables like broccoli, cauliflower and cabbage

- Lignans – bran, vegetables, sesame seeds and whole grains

- Zoochemicals —offal, fish and red meat. You can also get them from the plants that animals eat.

Antioxidants also include copper mineral which you can get from foods such as lean meat, nuts, and raw milk. Though lean meat is allowed, you should avoid all meat and processed meat products from non-organic sources as may be contaminated with hormones, antibiotics and pro inflammatory elements.

12. Observe the Budwig Protocol

The protocol was designed by a German expert on lipids and pharmacology, a globally acclaimed authority on fats and oils. Budwig discovered that majority of hydrogenated vegetable-based oils and other processed fats lead to toxicity in cells. The toxins are linked to diseases like cancer and other dangerous health complications among them the kidney disease.

But not all fats are bad and so the Budwig diet requires that you replace processed fats and oils with healthy fatty acids. But why are some fats considered healthy and others unhealthy?

Let's starts on the bad fats that Budwig protocol links to cell toxicity and precursor to cancer disease:

- **Trans Fats**

These are fats formed from chemical modification of other fats. Tran's fats usually go through a hydrogenation where the position of hydrogen in the fat molecule is adjusted. Though the process helps improve their shelf-life, consumption of these fats leads to higher cholesterol levels that may pose great danger to your health.

- **Polyunsaturated fat**

Despite being perceived as good sources of fats, these are highly processed and bad for your cell health. Studies have shown that liquid vegetable oil and trans-fats are linked to majority of the rising cancer and heart diseases. However, there's a distinction between natural polyunsaturated fat and processed polyunsaturated fat. Processed polyunsaturated fat is found on most of the margarines we spread on bread. The bad fats actually worsen HDL/LDL cholesterol levels and therefore are risky to your health. On the other hand, natural polyunsaturated fat helps in improving cholesterol levels and are good for your optimal health. You can get them from fatty fish, such as salmon, tuna and trout.

For the healthy fats options, you can adopt a few saturated fats and the mono-unsaturated fats.

- **Mono-unsaturated fats**

This type of fat has come to be widely accepted as healthy after a couple of research studies. Mono-unsaturated fats can help you achieve better insulin resistance levels and better HDL/LDL cholesterol levels, which are beneficial to your health. Examples of these fats include olive and sunflower oils.

- **Saturated fats**

Good news is that saturated fats are very necessary for your optimal health and poses no toxicity risk to health. These keep your immune levels at optimum levels, your bone density normal and testosterone levels in check. Foods that contain saturated fat include meat, eggs and butter, which help improve cholesterol levels.

Bugwig recommends consumption of healthy fats for variety of reasons. Some healthy fats also contain omega 3 fatty acids, which prevent inflammation and also boost heart and brain health. You can get omega-3 from flaxseeds, tuna sardines, herring, black cod and salmon. Also try to choose unsaturated fatty acids from products like flaxseed oil, flaxseeds and cottage cheese. Flax is rich in electron-rich unsaturated fatty acids while cottage cheese has saturated fats and sulfur proteins.

You can also adopt other healthy fats such as coconut oil. This oil serves as a potent source of Lauric acid, a heart healthy fatty acid that has antiviral and anti-bacterial properties that can help prevent cancer. Due to these factors, coconut oil is a great choice for boosting the immune system, through destruction of bacteria and viruses. For detox, coconut oil can help clean up the body, as it boosts its ability to process long chain fatty acids. The Lauric acid in the coconut oil is also in high amounts in breast milk, thus can work perfectly in supporting immune system in babies.

These fats when combined together can be easily absorbed into the body and supply necessary nutrients. Let's see a simple recipe that can help you obtain healthy fats and improve your condition:

- 1 tablespoon flaxseed oil

- 1/4 teaspoon black pepper

- 4 tablespoons sprouted and ground chia or flax

- 1 teaspoon turmeric powder

- 6 ounces cultured dairy say goat's milk kefir or cottage cheese

Combine these ingredients into a bowl or blend them into a drink.

With these tips or guidelines, no doubt you can easily adopt anti-inflammatory diet and successfully achieve your health objectives. And well, perhaps you may want some ideas on how an anti-inflammation meal should look like, right? In the next section, we shall look at how to get started on this diet for the first 7 days of your diet.

Here is a 1 week diet plan with suggestions on what foods to eat for breakfast, lunch, dinner and snacks.

7 Days Diet Plan

Day 1

Breakfast

Small palm-sized portion of macadamia nuts

Decaffeinated coffee

Snack

Smoked pork

Coconut cream

Homemade curried carrot soup

Lunch

Sauerkraut

Brown mustard

2 Poly-face uncured hot dogs

Snack

Hard boiled eggs

Diet gelatin with whipped cream

Cheese sticks

Dinner

Pureed cauliflower "rice"

Beef & broccoli with coconut aminos

Day 2

Breakfast

2 medium eggs cooked in bacon fat

1½ cup spinach

Snack

A fist full of kale chips, toast in salt, lemon zest and olive oil

Lunch

Homemade dijon vinaigrette

Smoked pork over green salad with carrots

Snack

Raw hazelnuts, broiled with tablespoon each of cocoa powder and coconut oil

Dinner

Black olives and fresh basil

Meatball salad with canned tomatoes

Day 3

Breakfast

2 over medium eggs

1.5 cups fresh spinach

1/4 lb Ground sausage

Snack

Canned tuna with 1/4 cup mayonnaise

Lunch

Leftover beef & broccoli

Dinner

Organ Meat Pie, made with ground beef, beef liver, carrots, broccoli and cauliflower puree.

Day 4:

Breakfast

Mushrooms

Caramelized onions

2 egg omelet

Snack

Buffalo jerky stick

Lunch

Coconut cream

Leftover organ meat pie

Homemade curried carrot soup

Snack

1/3 cup roasted, salted almonds

Dinner

1 fruit

2 tablespoons light dressing

4 ounces of chicken

A large Salad

Day 5:

Breakfast

Spinach and bacon

2 fried eggs

Snack

1/2 cup homemade salsa

Pork rinds

Lunch

Homemade dijon vinaigrette

A green salad

Tuna salad with homemade mayo

Snack

Palm full of macadamias

2 hard-boiled eggs

Dinner

Yellow squash

Grilled zucchini

Day 6

Breakfast

Decaffeinated Coffee

2 hardboiled eggs

Snack

30g mixed dried fruit

10 cashews

Lunch

1/3 chicken breast without dressing

Green salad

Snack

Lettuce, tomato and mustard

5-guys bun-less burger

Dinner

Roasted zucchini and yellow squash

Diced tomatoes

Venison meatloaf

Day 7:

Breakfast

Egg salad

1/2 avocado

Carrot sticks

Decaffeinated coffee

Snack

Palm full of macadamia nuts

Lunch

1/2 cup cauliflower salad

1 1/2 chicken thigh

1 1/2 pork backbones

Snack

Sausages

Leftover eggs salad

Dinner

A green salad

Sliced flank steak

Drizzled balsamic vinegar

It's recommended that you cook your own meals as buying pre-packaged food may subject you to unhealthy foods or processed ingredients. Though you may not enjoy cooking, you can begin from simple recipes such as steamed veggies and sticky rice served with hot spices.

Running out of ideas? Well, here is a comprehensive list of over 40 recipes that you can prepare at any time of the day. They have been categorized into breakfast, main dishes and snacks and desserts to help you easily find them.

Anti-Inflammatory Recipes

Breakfast Recipes

Buckwheat and Quinoa Granola

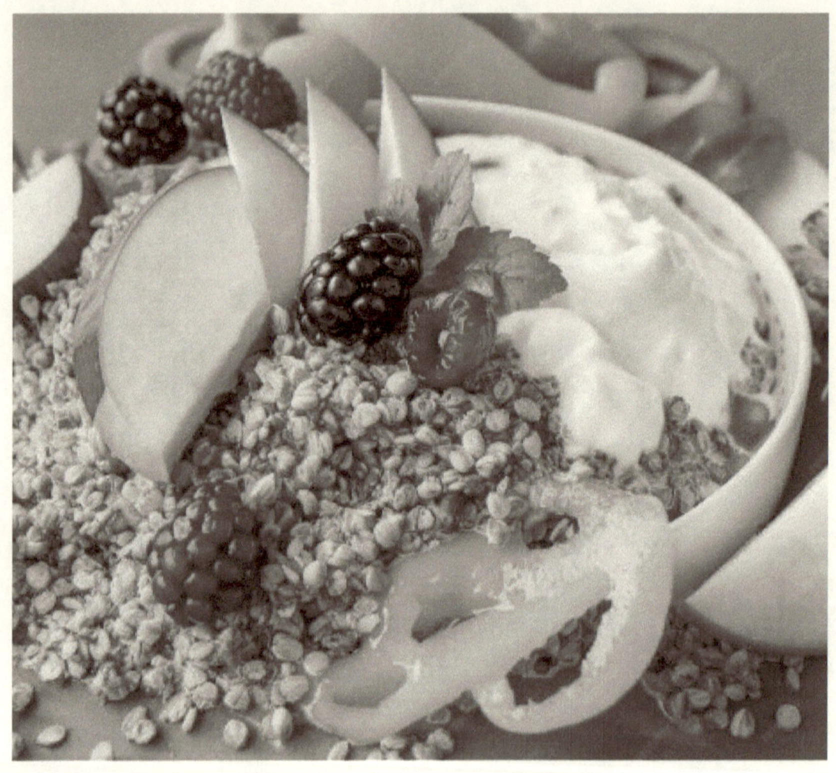

Serves 6

Ingredients

A piece of ginger

4 tablespoons of raw cacao powder

6 tablespoons of coconut oil

1 cup of apple puree/sauce

1 and ½ cups of pitted dates

1 cup of pumpkin seeds

1 cup of sunflower seeds

1 cup of buckwheat

2 cups of oats

Directions

1. Preheat your oven to 180 degrees Celsius. Then on a baking sheet, line silicon baking mat or parchment paper.

2. In a large bowl, stir together oats, quinoa and buckwheat. Set aside.

3. In a small bowl or saucepan, stir together apple puree, coconut oil and dates. Now simmer for around 5 minutes to soften the dates.

4. Meanwhile, peel the ginger and grate into a bowl. Mix it into the pan with cooking dates.

5. Put the cooked dates, apple puree, grated ginger and melted coconut oil in a blender along with cacao powder.

6. Puree to smoothness then pour the mixture over the oat and buckwheat mixture. Stir well to evenly coat the mixture.

7. Once the mixture is fully blended, spread into a prepared pan to make an even layer.

8. Bake the mixture in the preheated oven for around 40 or 45 minutes.

7. Remove the trays from the oven after approximately 15 minutes and stir the mixture to ensure the top doesn't burn. Repeat this step every 5-10 minutes until the granola is cooked through.

8. Once it's well cooked and crispy, transfer the granola to a cooling rack to completely cool down, and then store in an airtight container.

Rhubarb, Apple and Ginger Muffin

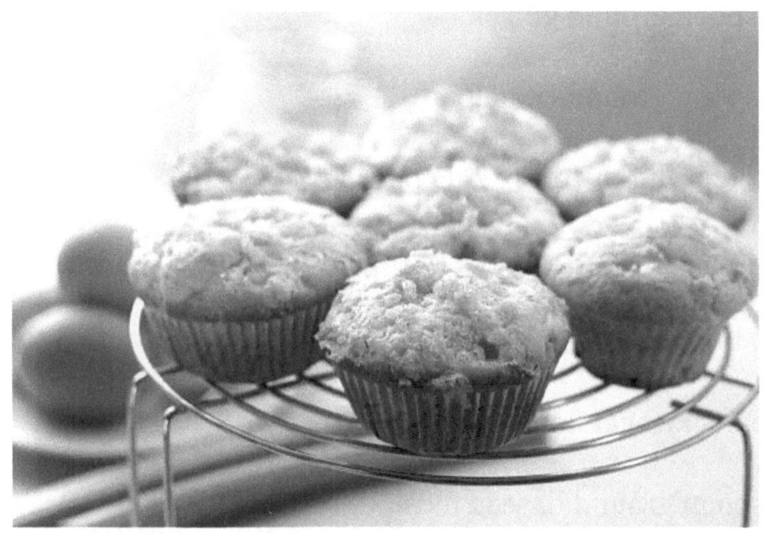

Serves 8

Ingredients

1 teaspoon vanilla extract

1 large free-range egg

1/4 cup olive oil

95 ml rice or almond milk

1 small apple, peeled, cored and finely diced

1 cup rhubarb, finely sliced

Sea salt to taste

1/2 teaspoon ground ginger

1/2 teaspoon ground cinnamon

2 teaspoons gluten-free baking powder

2 tablespoons true arrowroot or organic corn flour

1/4 cup brown rice flour

1/2 cup buckwheat flour

1 tablespoon ground linseed meal

2 tablespoons crystallized ginger, finely chopped

1/4 cup unrefined raw sugar

1/2 cup ground almonds or almond meal

Directions

1. Preheat oven to 350 degrees F. Meanwhile lightly grease or line 8 1/3-cup capacity muffin pan or tins with paper liners.

2. In a medium-sized bowl, whisk together linseed meal, ginger, sugar and almond meal.

3. Sieve the mixture over flours, spices and baking powder. Whisk the contents to incorporate.

4. Now stir in the apple and rhubarb to coat the flour mixture. In a separate bowl, whisk vanilla, egg, oil and milk then pour into the dry mixture. Stir to fully mix.

5. Divide the batter between paper cases or tins then scatter rhubarb slices.

6. Bake in the preheated oven for 20 to 25 minutes or until its golden around the edges. When you insert a toothpick at the center, it should come out clean.

7. Remove from the oven and cool for 5 minutes. Then move to a wire rack until cool enough to handle.

8. Serve it warm or cool. You can store frozen in zip-lock bags or an airtight container until ready to serve.

Amaranth Porridge

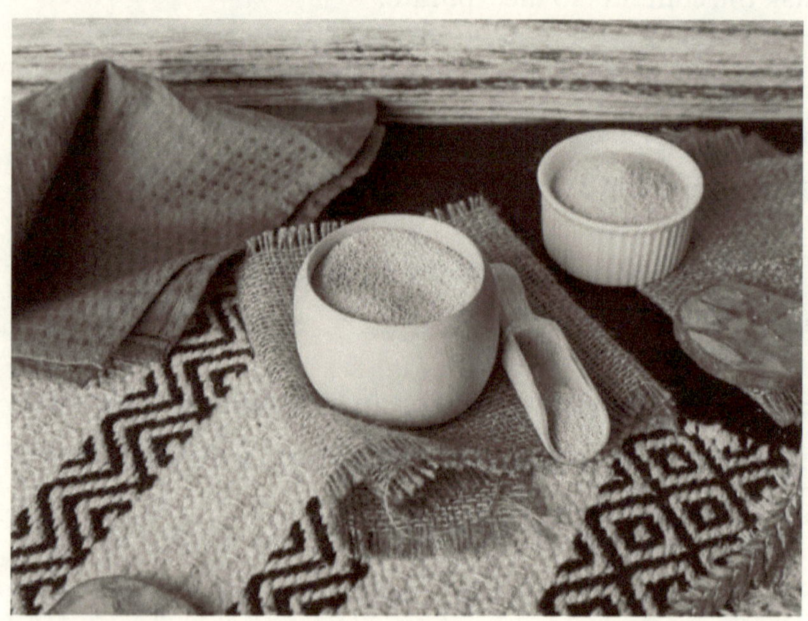

Serves: 2

Ingredients

1 medium pear, chopped

½ cup blueberries or cranberries, dried

1 teaspoon cinnamon

1 tablespoon raw honey

¼ cup hemp or pumpkin seeds

2 cup filtered water

2/3 cup whole-grain amaranth

Directions

1. In a skillet or a heavy 2-quart saucepan, mix together amaranth and water and close with a tight fitting lid. Ensure you stir the porridge constantly to prevent sticking.

2. Bring the amaranth mixture to a boil, cover and then lower the heat to simmer for around 25-30 minutes. Keep stirring at 10 minutes interval to ensure that the grains don't stick to pot.

3. As soon as the water is fully absorbed, remove the porridge from heat and then add in cinnamon, raw honey and the seeds, and then stir well.

4. Now divide the porridge among two bowls, or keep a portion in a sealable container to serve next day. Top with pears and blueberries if you like.

Gluten-Free Oatmeal

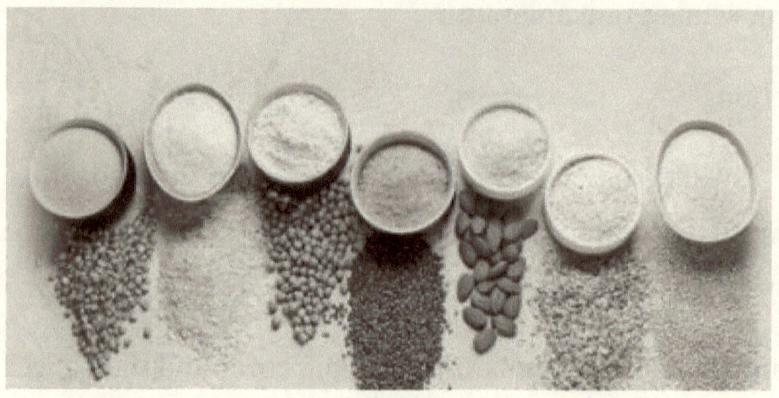

Serves 2

Ingredients

1 cup whole rolled gluten-free oats

1 teaspoon vanilla extract

1/2 teaspoon kosher salt

1 cup water

1 cup whole milk, almond milk or hemp milk

Directions

1. Over high heat, pour water and milk in a sauce pan then add in vanilla extract and salt. Bring the mixture to a boil.

2. As the liquids boil, pour in gluten-free oats. Stir to mix. After the liquids begin to boil again, lower the heat to simmer the oats while stirring occasionally.

3. Cook for about 15 minutes (make sure that the oats are nicely creamy and fairly plump and the liquid mixture is completely absorbed).

4. At this point, turn off the heat and then proceed to cover the sauce pan. Allow the oatmeal to cool for around 5 minutes.

5. Then top with preferred fruits such as blackberries and peaches.

Spanish Frittata

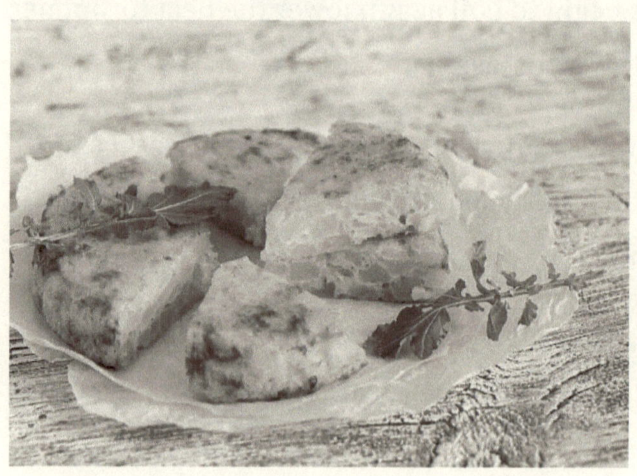

Serves 4-6

1 cup of arugula or spinach

½ cup sautéed mushrooms

1 small red onion, finely chopped

2 tablespoons extra-virgin olive oil or coconut oil

½ teaspoon sea salt

½ cup coconut milk

12 large organic eggs

Directions

1. First preheat your oven to 375 degrees F. Meanwhile, whisk coconut milk, eggs and 2 pinches of salt. Then set the mixture aside.

2. Over medium heat, prepare a pan with coconut or extra virgin olive oil and sauté the onions for about 3 minutes, or until translucent.

3. Add in the mushrooms or other vegetable and sauté until it's soft. Toss in the spinach and then fold into the veggie mixture to wilt. Once it's done, remove the pan and now set aside.

4. Lower the heat and add more coconut oil if needed. In the same skillet, add in the eggs and shake to distribute and then cook for 5 minutes over medium low heat.

5. Use a spatula to spread the eggs from edges to center up until the edges are no longer runny. Then arrange the vegetable mixture and top over evenly.

6. At this point, move the mixture into an oven and cook for around 5 minutes or until lightly browned, and then remove from the oven.

7. Slide the cooked frittata partially onto a large plate, and place a plate over the pan using oven mitts. Then hold the

plate and pan and invert them to make the frittata drop into the plate.

8. Now slide the frittata into the pan with the partially cooked side facing up.

9. Return in the oven and continue to cook for about 3-4 minutes, and then serve over simple salad with citrus vinaigrette.

Portobello Breakfast Bakes

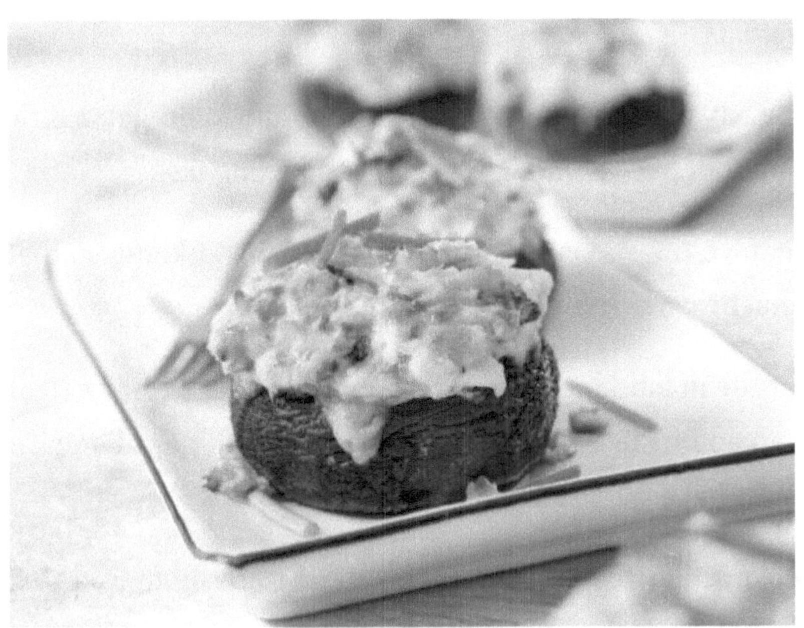

Serves 2

Ingredients:

Salt & pepper

2 tablespoons parsley, chopped

4 slices bacon

2-4 large eggs

2 Portobello mushroom caps

1 tablespoon coconut oil or olive oil

Directions

1. Preheat your oven to 400 degrees F and then get a little coconut or olive oil and lightly grease a baking dish.

2. Remove the stems from mushrooms using a knife, so that the mushrooms attain a small bowl shape.

3. Put the mushroom cups into the baking dish with the right side up and bake for about 5 minutes. Then flip upside down and now bake for another 5 minutes.

4. Meanwhile, prepare the bacon. Using an aluminum foil, line a baking sheet and then position the bacon strips in a single layer of the baking sheet.

6. Bake the bacon for 10-15 minutes until done. Once done, remove the caps from heat and then crack 1-2 eggs in each; and return the mushrooms and eggs into the oven.

6. At this point, bake these for additional 10-15 minutes for the egg whites and yolks to be cooked as you like them to be.

7. Then let the bacon to cool down before cutting it into bite sizes. To serve, sprinkle the bacon bits and eggs with parsley.

Hash with Poached Eggs

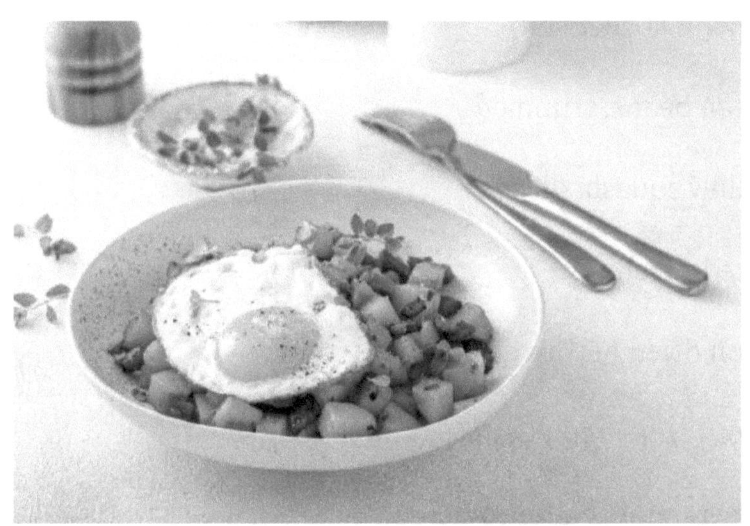

Serves 4

Ingredients

1 ounce Parmesan cheese, shredded

4 large eggs

1 tablespoon white vinegar

2 tablespoons fresh parsley, chopped

2 tablespoons chives, thinly sliced

2 cups seeded tomato, chopped

1/2 teaspoon black pepper, ground

1/2 teaspoon kosher salt

1 cup green beans, trimmed

1 cup yellow squash, diced

1 cup diced zucchini

1 teaspoon dried herbes de Provence

1 cup sliced small red potatoes or fingerling

1 cup sweet onion, chopped

4 teaspoons olive oil

Directions

1. Over medium heat, warm a large non-stick skillet and add in oil, and then swirl to coat.

2. Now add in herbes de Provence, potatoes and onions, and then spread the mixture in a single layer. Cook without stirring for 4 minutes, to have the potatoes lightly turn brown.

3. Then lower the heat to medium and now stir in 3/8 spoon pepper, salt, beans, yellow squash and zucchini.

4. When ready, remove from heat and cover the pan, and then allow it to rest for 5 minutes. Then stir in the parsley, chives and tomato.

5. To a large skillet, add in water up to 2/3rd full and bring it to a boil. Then lower the heat to simmer, and then stir in vinegar.

6. Now in a custard cup, break each of the 4 eggs and then pour gently into the pan.

7. Cook for around 3 minutes, and then use a slotted spoon to remove the eggs from the pan.

8. At this point, sub-divide the mixture into 4 plates and top each with an egg.

9. You can use the remaining Parmesan cheese and 1/8 teaspoon pepper to sprinkle on eggs.

Cinnamon Baked Apples

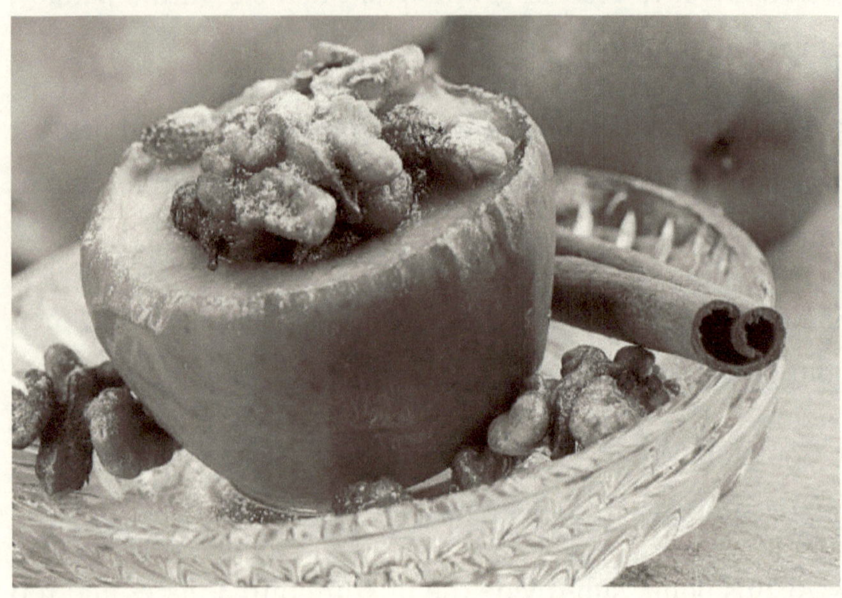

Serves: 4

Ingredients

1 cup apple juice or cider

¼ cup liquid honey, unpasteurized

4 apples

¼ teaspoon ground cloves

½ teaspoon nutmeg

1 teaspoon cinnamon

1 teaspoon grated fresh ginger root

2 dates, pitted and chopped

¼ cup dried cranberries

½ cup nuts and/or seeds

Directions

1. Preheat your oven to 325 degrees F and then combine spices, ginger root, dates, cranberries and nuts and seeds in a bowl.

2. Core out the core of the apples, without peeling. It's important to do so as most nutrients and fiber are found on the skin.

3. Stuff each apple using the seed and nut mixture and then drizzle some honey. Put the batter into an 8 x 8 inch square baking dish.

4. Pour in the juice around the apple to keep it moist, and then bake in the preheated oven for around 30-35 minutes.

5. As soon as the apples are soft, remove from the oven and serve.

Lunch Recipes

Quinoa Salad with Cashews

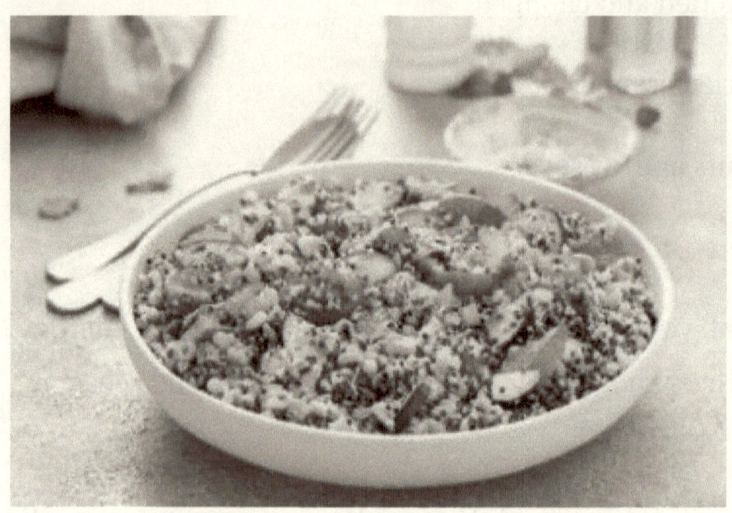

Serves 4

Ingredients

3 cups Romaine lettuce, chopped

1 cup cashews, coarsely chopped

1 avocado, chopped or thinly sliced

½-inch-piece ginger, finely chopped

Black pepper, freshly ground

1 teaspoon sea salt, to taste

¼ cup mint, finely chopped

1 large mango, chopped

1 tablespoon extra-virgin olive oil

2 tablespoons honey or agave

Juice of 1 lime

1 cup apple or carrot, finely chopped

½ red onion, finely chopped

1 cup dried quinoa, rinsed well

Directions

1. First cook the quinoa. To cook, simply bring to boil 2 cups of water in a saucepan then add quinoa.

2. Cover and simmer for around 15-20 minutes. Once cooked through, set aside and allow to cool.

3. Now toss apple or carrot with chopped onions in a large bowl. In a separate bowl, whisk together olive oil, honey and lime juice and add the mixture to the bowl.

4. Then add in cooked quinoa and mango and toss to mix. Add in ginger, cilantro, mint, pepper and salt.

5. Garnish with cashews and sliced avocado. To serve, scoop the mixture over the greens.

Mediterranean Fish

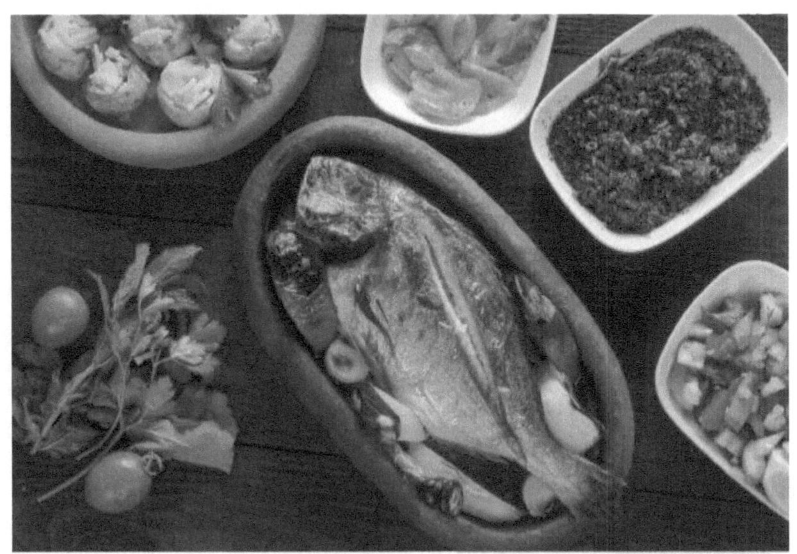

Serves 4

Ingredients

Salt and pepper

1 tablespoon lemon juice

1/4 cup olive oil

1/4 cup capers

5 ounce pitted kalamata olives

1 onion, chopped

1 large tomato, chopped

1 tablespoon Greek seasoning

4-6 ounce fillets halibut

Directions

1. First preheat your oven to 350 F degrees.

2. Then put the halibut fillets on an aluminum foil and use Greek seasoning to season.

3. Now mix together pepper, salt, lemon juice, olive oil, capers, olives, onion and tomatoes in a bowl.

4. At this point, spoon the tomato onion mixture over the fish, then seal all the edges using a foil to create a large packet.

5. On a baking sheet, put the packet and bake it in the preheated oven for about 30 to 40 minutes.

6. Once the halibut can flake easily, remove from the oven and serve.

Honey Roasted Carrots with Thyme

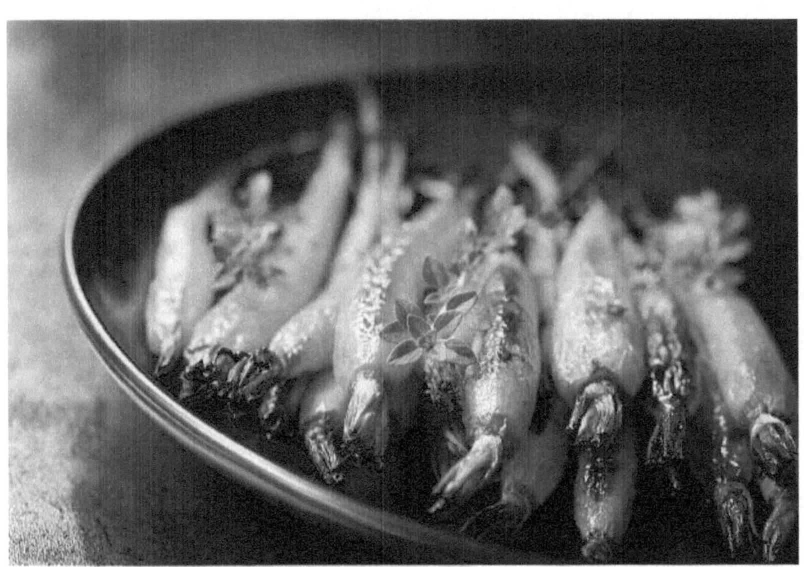

Serves 4

Ingredients

1 teaspoon fresh thyme or ½ teaspoon dried thyme

½ teaspoon sea salt

1 tablespoon raw honey

2 tablespoons olive oil

1 large bunch carrots, scrubbed

Directions

1. First preheat your oven to 425 degrees F. Meanwhile, line a baking sheet with parchment paper.

2. Then toss the carrots with thyme, salt, honey and oil. Arrange the ingredients in an even layer and bake for 30 minutes.

3. Remove from the oven as soon as it has browned and caramelized and let cool for a moment. Serve and enjoy.

Beet the Detox Salad

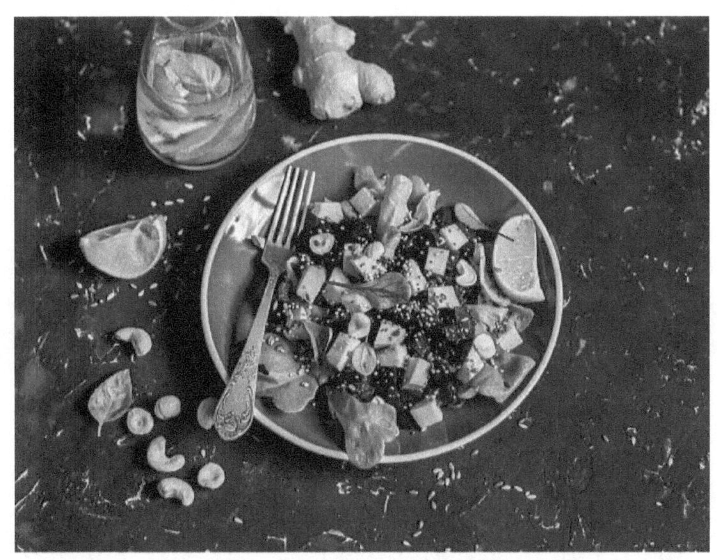

Servings: 4

Ingredients

4 cups of mixed greens

2 tablespoons of lemon juice

2 tablespoons flax, pumpkin, hemp or seed oil

2 tablespoons almonds, chopped

1 large apple, diced

1 large carrot, coarsely grated

1 large beet, coarsely grated

Optional

1/4 teaspoon gray sea salt or pink rock salt

2 garlic cloves, minced

2 tablespoons fresh dill or parsley, finely chopped

Directions

1. In a large bowl, toss all the other ingredients apart from the mixed greens.

2. Then add in the optional add-ons if you like it. Alternatively, you can prepare the dressing 2 days in advance and keep in the fridge.

3. Divide the salad greens between 4 plates and top with the apple mixture if you like it.

Sesame Shrimp Stir Fry with Veggies

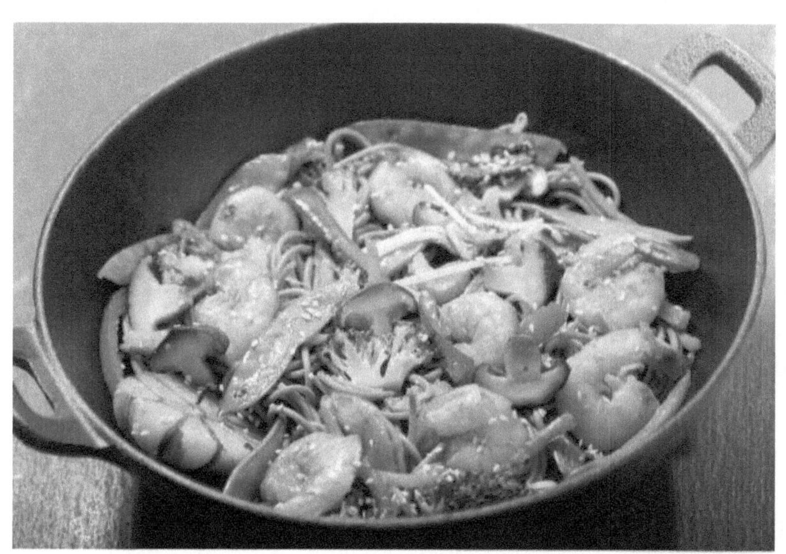

Serves 4

Ingredients

2 cups rainbow chard, thinly sliced

2 garlic cloves minced

3 ounces shitake mushrooms, thinly sliced

1 small yellow squash cut into matchsticks

1 bell pepper seeded and sliced

1 small yellow onion, halved and thinly sliced

1 pound large wild shrimp, peeled and deveined

2 tablespoons coconut oil, divided

2 tablespoons shelled hemp seed, organic

2 tablespoons raw honey

2 teaspoons sesame oil

¼ cup liquid aminos or soy sauce

Directions

1. Whisk together hemp seeds, raw honey, sesame oil and liquid aminos in a mixing bowl.

2. In a large non-stick skillet or a wok, heat a tablespoon of coconut oil. Add shrimp and stir-fry for 2 minutes on high heat. As soon as it's no longer pink, move to a bowl and set aside.

3. Now add the remaining oil and stir-fry the shitakes, squash, peppers and onion for 5 minutes, or until lightly charred.

4. Then add in garlic and cook for a minute, or until fragrant. Stir in chard and cook for about 2 minutes, or until wilted.

5. Add the sauce and simmer for 2 more minutes, or until it thickens slightly. Finally fold in the shrimp and cook for a minute.

6. Serve the fish and veggies over quinoa or brown rice.

Root Vegetable Tagine with Kale

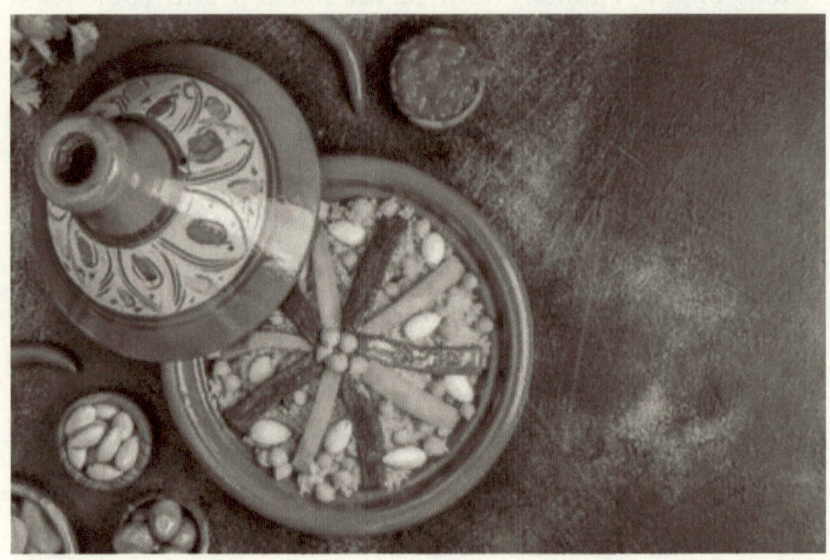

Serves 6

Ingredients

¼ cup cilantro leaves roughly chopped

2 tablespoons lemon juice

2 cups kale leaves, roughly chopped

1 quart vegetable stock

2 medium diced carrots or 2 bunches baby carrots, peeled

2 medium purple potatoes, peeled and diced

2 medium sweet potatoes peeled and diced

3 tablespoons of tomato paste

1 teaspoon sea salt

2 large cloves garlic minced

¼ teaspoon cayenne pepper

½ teaspoon ground cinnamon

½ teaspoon ground ginger

1 teaspoon ground cumin

1 medium parsnip peeled and diced

1 large sweet onion diced

2 tablespoons olive or coconut oil

Slivered almonds, toasted

Directions

1. Heat oil in a Dutch oven or large stock pot. Over medium high heat, sauté the onion for 5 minutes or until soft then add in parsnip.

2. Cook for 3 minutes or until golden brown. Stir in tomato paste, cayenne, salt, cinnamon, ginger, ground cumin and garlic.

3. Cook for 2 minutes or until very fragrant then fold in carrots, purple potatoes and sweet potatoes.

4. Add vegetable stock and bring to a boil, then lower the heat to medium-low.

5. Simmer uncovered for around 20 minutes or until veggies are tender, while stirring after every few minutes.

6. Then stir in lemon juice and kale, and simmer until the leaves are vibrant and slightly wilted, in about 2 minutes.

7. Garnish the dish with nuts and cilantro if you like. Serve over conscious or quinoa.

Kale and Fruit Salad

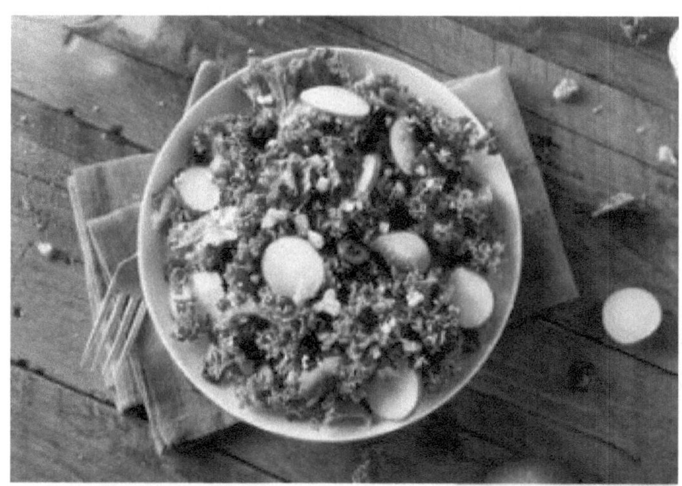

Serves 2-3

Ingredients for the salad:

1/2 a red onion, very thinly sliced

2 bunches kale, or 6 packed cups of baby kale

6 Medjool dates, pitted

1/3 cup whole hazelnuts

For the dressing

5 tablespoons toasted hazelnut oil

Pinch of coarse salt

1 Medjool date

4 tablespoons orange juice, freshly squeezed

2 tablespoons Apple Cider Vinegar

Directions

1. First preheat your oven to 375 degrees F. Meanwhile, put hazelnuts in a baking dish and roast until the skin darkens and start to split, or for approximately 7-8 minutes.

2. Then move the nuts while still hot to steam for another 15 minutes while wrapped in a kitchen towel. This helps remove the skin from the nuts.

3. Once cool enough, squeeze and twist around firmly to remove the skin, but while still wrapped into towel.

4. In a food processor, put the hazelnuts and pulse them until fully mixed and finely chopped. Set it aside to top the salad.

5. Wash, dry and chop the kales and then put into a large bowl. Slice the onion thinly and add into the bowl.

6. Prepare the dressing by combining the ingredients for dressing in the blender apart from the oil.

7. Puree the mixture to break down the dates and then drizzle the oil in a steady stream to emulsify the dressing.

8. At this point, toss the kale and onion mixture along with the orange-hazel nut dressing together.

9. Then move to a platter bowl and sprinkle with the hazelnut and dates mixture.

Raw Pad Thai

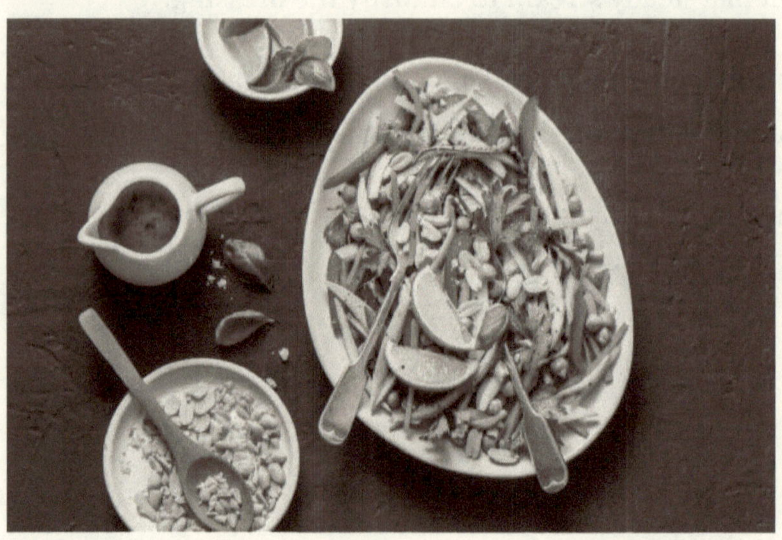

Serves: 4

Ingredients

½ cup radish sprouts or bean sprouts

½ cup cauliflower florets

½ cup shredded purple cabbage

1 green onion, chopped

1 large carrot

1 medium zucchini

For Sauce:

½ teaspoon ginger root, grated

¼ teaspoon garlic, minced

1 tablespoon raw honey

2 tablespoons tamari (wheat-free)

1 tablespoon lime or lemon juice

2 tablespoons almond butter

2 tablespoons tahini

Directions

1. Using a vegetable peeler or mandolin, make noodles from zucchini and carrots.

2. Then put the ingredients into a large mixing bowl and then top with the veggies.

3. In a bowl, whisk the sauce ingredients to obtain a thick mixture, which will thin out when combined with veggies.

4. Now pour the sauce over the veggies and noodles and toss. The meal is even sweeter next day as flavors are fully incorporated.

Dinner Recipes

Salmon and Quinoa Bowls with Yogurt Sauce

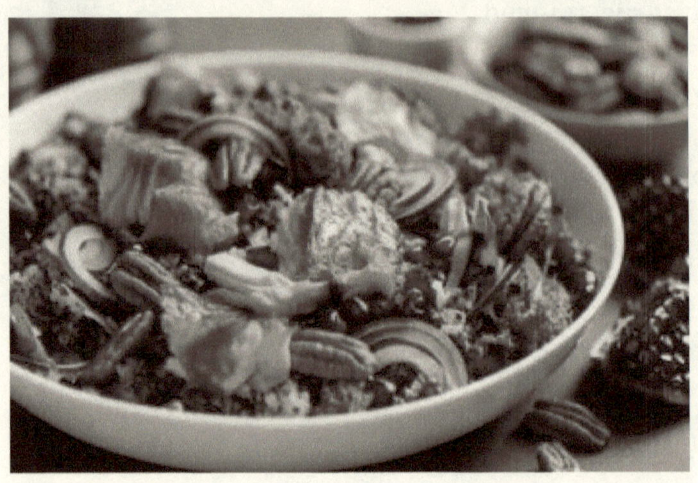

Serves 4

Ingredients

1/4 cup dried currants, cranberries or cherries

2 cups cooked chickpeas, rinsed and drained

Sea salt

Olive oil

2 garlic cloves, minced

2 tablespoons lemon juice

1 medium carrot, peeled and thinly sliced

1 bunch dinosaur kale, thinly sliced

1 cup white quinoa

Four 4-ounce sockeye salmon fillets

1 tablespoon hemp seeds

For the sauce:

1/2 teaspoon sea salt

1/2 cup Greek yogurt

1 tablespoon lemon juice

1/2 cup water

1/4 cup tahini paste

Directions

1. Mix together 2 cups of water and quinoa in a medium saucepan.

2. Bring to a boil, cover and set the heat to low. Cook for around 15 minutes then let cook 10 minutes off the heat. Set aside.

3. Mix together sea salt, 2 tablespoons olive oil, garlic, lemon juice, carrots and kale in a large mixing bowl.

4. Toss the kales with your hands until well coated in oil and lemon. Add the cooked quinoa along with hemp seeds, dried fruits and chickpeas. Mix well to blend then adjust the seasoning as desired.

5. In a cast iron skillet or non-stick skillet, heat 2 tablespoons of oil. Pat the fish dry and season with some salt.

6. Cook the fish over high heat skin-side down for about 2-3 minutes, or until nicely browned. Flip the salmon and cook until its opaque up the sides, in 2 minutes or so.

7. Divide the quinoa between serving plates and top with seared fish. Then whisk together sauce ingredients in a mixing bowl.

8. Add water to the smooth mixture to make it easier to drizzle. Spoon the sauce over the salmon and serve.

Sweet Potato Burgers and Black Bean

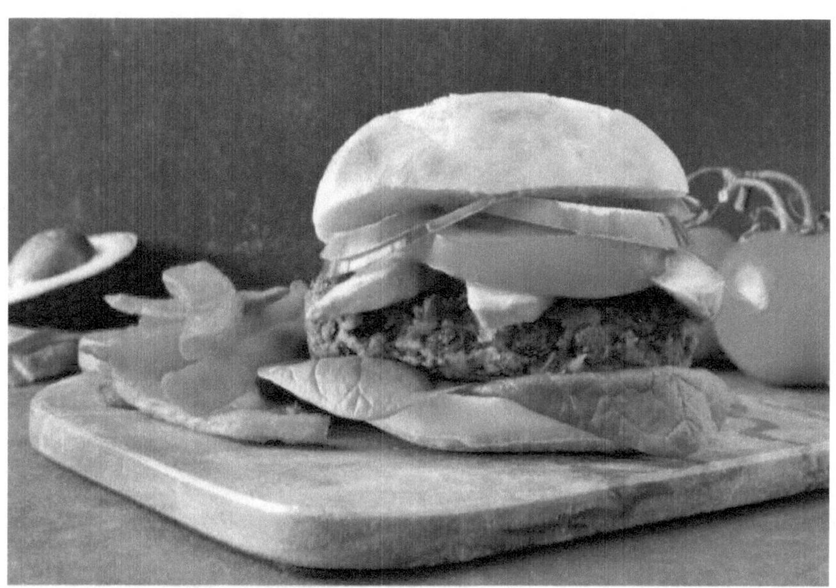

Serves: 8

Ingredients

Hamburger buns, whole wheat

1 cup plain breadcrumbs, divided

2 eggs, lightly beaten

2 ½ cups raw sweet potato, grated

3 cups black beans, drained, rinsed and mashed

3 teaspoons minced garlic

2 teaspoons ground cumin

1 jalapeno, minced

1 medium-sized onion, chopped

Vegetable cooking spray

½ teaspoon hot sauce

2 lime

½ cup reduced fat mayonnaise

Directions

1. Over medium heat, preheat your broiler and then set the oven rack about 4-5 inches from the broiler.

2. In small bowl, zest and squeeze the lime and then add hot sauce and mayonnaise. Stir to fully blend and then put into the fridge until you need to serve.

3. Spray a large skillet with cooking spray and then heat over medium heat. Add in onions and cook until tender, for about 3-4 minutes.

4. Then stir in garlic, cumin, jalapeno and continue to cook for 30 more seconds.

5. Pour the onion mixture in a separate bowl and add in ½ cup breadcrumbs, egg, sweet potato and mashed black beans. Stir to fully combine.

6. Make 8 patties from the mixture and then use the remaining ½ cup of breadcrumbs to sprinkle on the patties.

7. Once done, put the patties on a baking sheet that is lightly greased with cooking spray.

8. Bake the patties for 10-20 minutes each side until cooked through and golden brown.

9. Serve the meal hot over lime mayonnaise and hamburger buns.

Fried Rice with Snap Peas and Scallions

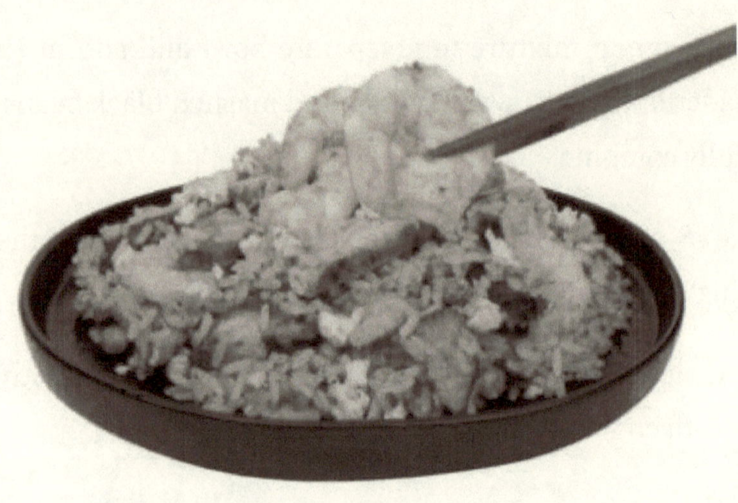

Serves 4

Ingredients

1 tablespoon shelled hemp seed, organic

2 eggs beaten

1 teaspoon sriracha

2 teaspoons toasted sesame oil

3 tablespoons liquid aminos

3 cups cooked black rice from 1 cup uncooked

1 tablespoon fresh ginger, minced

2 garlic cloves minced

1 cup thinly sliced snap peas

1 bunch scallions, thinly sliced

1 small yellow onion diced

2 medium carrots diced

2 tablespoons organic coconut oil

Directions

1. Heat coconut oil in a non-stick skillet or large wok. Sauté white scallion, onion and carrot over medium heat for about 5 minutes, or until soft and starts to brown.

2. Add in green scallions, ginger, garlic and snap peas then stir fry for 2 minutes, or until fragrant.

3. Fold in rice and stir fry for another 2 minutes, or until well-coated and starts to toast. Add in sriracha, sesame oil and liquid aminos and stir to mix.

4. At this point, push the rice to the side of the pan to make a well. Pour eggs in the center. Cook until nearly set while stirring.

5. Toss the rice with eggs and hemp seeds then move the rice to serving bowls.

Spice-Rubbed Bison Tenderloin

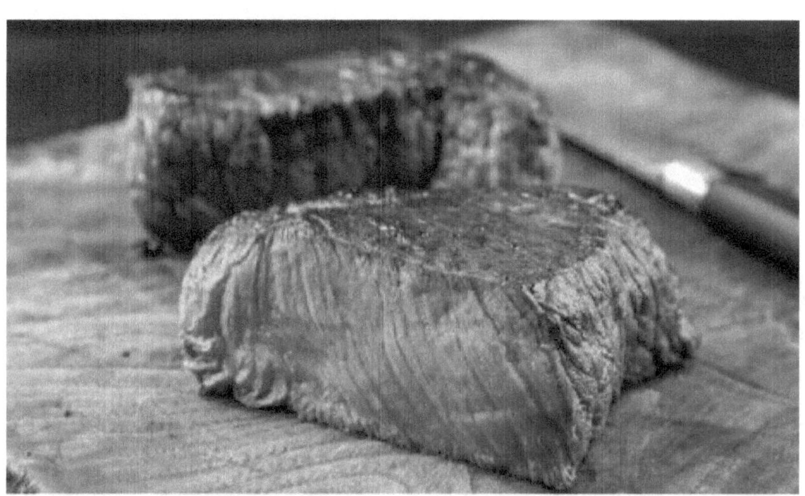

Serves: 4

Ingredients

4 six-ounce bison or beef tenderloin filets

½ teaspoon gray sea salt or pink rock salt

1 teaspoon minced fresh ginger root

½ teaspoon allspice

2 teaspoons cumin seeds, dry-toasted and ground

2 teaspoons coriander seeds, ground

1 teaspoon cinnamon

2 tablespoons minced garlic

2 sprigs fresh rosemary

Directions

1. Mix together ginger root, spices, garlic and rosemary in a small bowl and set aside.

2. Put the bison or beef on a 12 x 12 inch glass baking dish, and then coat both sides using the spice mix.

3. Now preheat the broiler on low and then put the fillets under it, around 6 inches from heat. Use medium low heat if using a grill pan on a stove.

4. Drizzle the meat with broth or filtered water to keep it moist. This also ensures your spices don't catch fire.

5. Grill or broil for around 4 to 6 minutes until done, while checking the meat not to overcook it.

6. As soon as it's done, remove from the grill or oven and allow to cool. Serve and enjoy.

Prosciutto-Wrapped Basil Shrimp

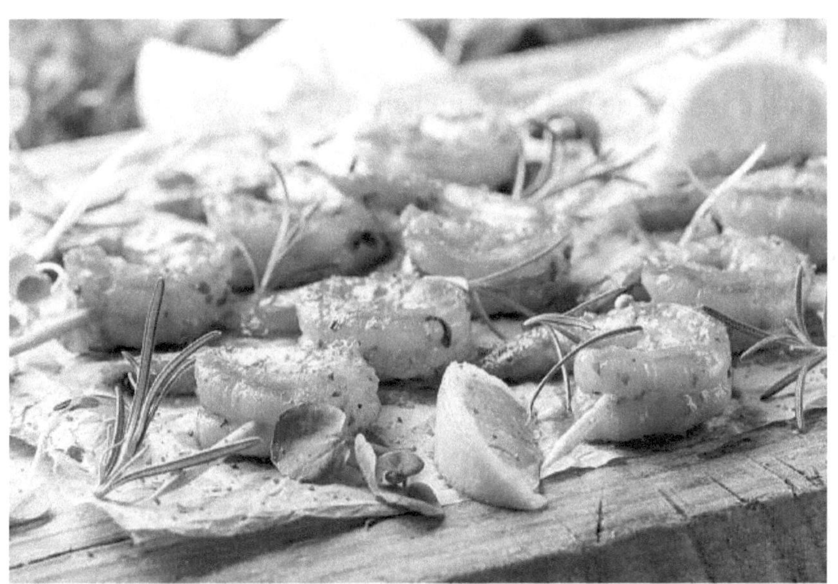

Serves 4

Ingredients

10 very thin slices prosciutto

1/8 teaspoon black pepper, freshly ground

1/4 teaspoon red pepper flakes

1/2 teaspoon kosher salt

1/2 teaspoon lemon zest

1 teaspoon extra-virgin olive oil

1 tablespoon fresh basil, chopped

20 large frozen peeled deveined shrimp, thawed

8 lemon wedges, optional

Cooking spray

Directions

1. First preheat the broiler.

2. Then mix together black pepper, red pepper flakes, salt, zest, olive oil, basil and shrimp. Combine well and set aside.

3. On a large work surface, lay the prosciutto slices then cut each into half lengthwise.

4. Then wrap the prosciutto pieces around each shrimp, but leave the tail hanging out.

5. Thread the shrimp on an 8-inch skewer and repeat the process for the rest of the shrimp to make 4 skewers with 5 shrimp each.

6. Put the skewers on a broiling pan that is greased with cooking spray. Broil the prosciutto-wrapped shrimp for about 2 minutes on each side.

7. Serve the dish hot with lemon wedges if you like.

Black-Bean Chili with Winter Squash

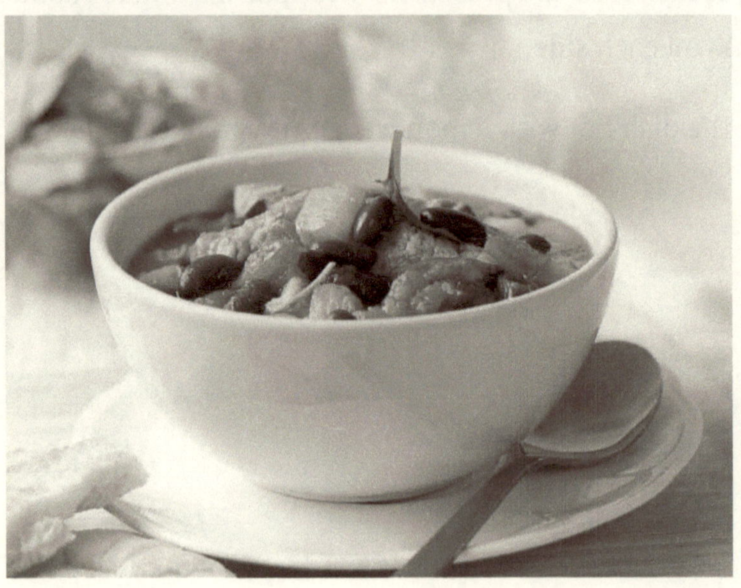

Serves 6

Ingredients

1/4 teaspoon salt

1 medium winter squash

1/2 teaspoon dried oregano

1 /4 teaspoon chipotle chile powder

1 teaspoon chili powder

1 (4.5-ounce) can mild green chiles, chopped

1 (28-ounce) can diced tomatoes, un-drained

2 cups fat-free, less-sodium vegetable broth

2 (15-ounce) cans black beans, rinsed and drained

3 garlic cloves, minced

1 medium yellow bell pepper, diced

1 large chopped onion

1 tablespoon olive oil

Directions

1. Over medium heat, add oil, onion and bell pepper and cook for about 5 minutes, stirring often.

2. Once soft, add in garlic and cook for another minute. Stir in oregano, chipotle powder, chili powder, green chiles, tomatoes, broth and beans.

3. Simmer for 10 minutes while covered. Then uncover and cook for another 10 minutes.

4. Now cut the squash in half, remove the seeds then pierce with a fork a number of times. Place in a heat-proof dish along with ¼ inch water.

5. Using plastic wrap, cover with and microwave on high until tender, or for 8 minutes.

6. Then allow to cool until safe to handle. Use a small sharp knife to peel the squash and cut into ½ inch chunks.

7. Stir the squash chunks into the bean mixture and cook for about 5 minutes. Season with salt and serve warm.

Poached Eggs with Curried Potatoes

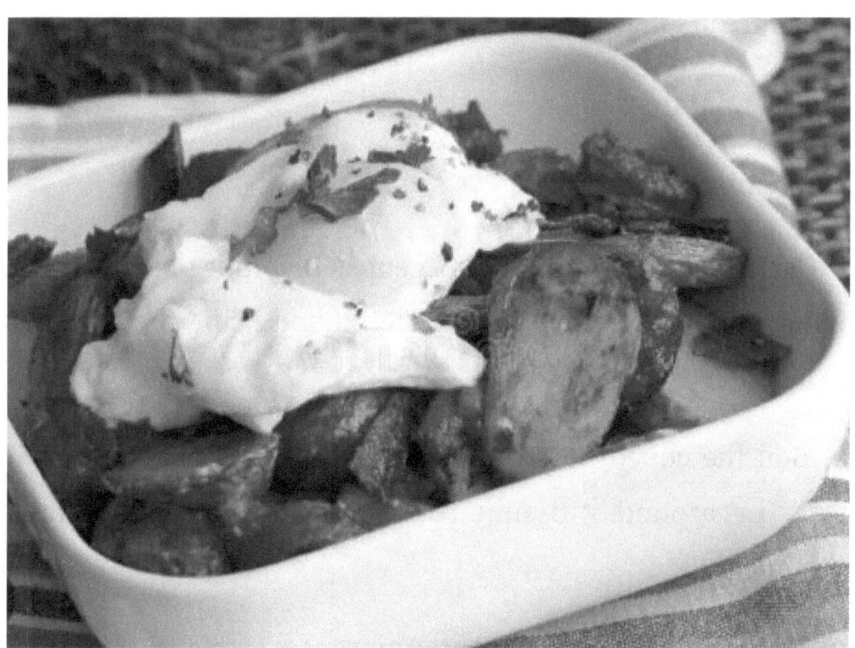

Serves: 4

Ingredients

½ bunch fresh cilantro

4 large eggs

1 15 oz. can tomato sauce

2 tablespoons curry powder

1 tablespoon olive oil

2 cloves garlic

1 inch fresh ginger

2 russet potatoes

Directions

1. Cut the potatoes into ¾ inch cubes then put the cubes in a pot. Cover with water, put on the lid and bring the potatoes to a boil over high heat.

2. Boil the cubed potatoes until tender when pierced with a fork, or around 5-6 minutes. Drain and put them in a colander.

3. Meanwhile, start to prepare the sauce. Using the side of a spoon of vegetable peeler, peel the skin off from ginger and then grate about 1 inch of ginger with a small holed cheese grater.

4. Mince the garlic then put in a large deep skillet. Add in olive oil and garlic then sauté over medium low heat until soft and fragrant, in about 1-2 minutes.

5. To the skillet, add curry powder and sauté for a minute to toast the spices. Then add in tomato sauce and stir to blend.

6. Set the heat to medium for the sauce to heat through. Taste and adjust the salt as needed.

7. Then add the drained potatoes and stir to coat with the sauce. If need be, add a few tablespoons of water.

8. At this point, make 4 dips or wells in the potato mixture and crack the egg into each. Put the lid on and simmer for around 6-10 minutes or until cooked through.

9. Top the meal with chopped fresh cilantro.

Vegan Garlic Sesame Noodles

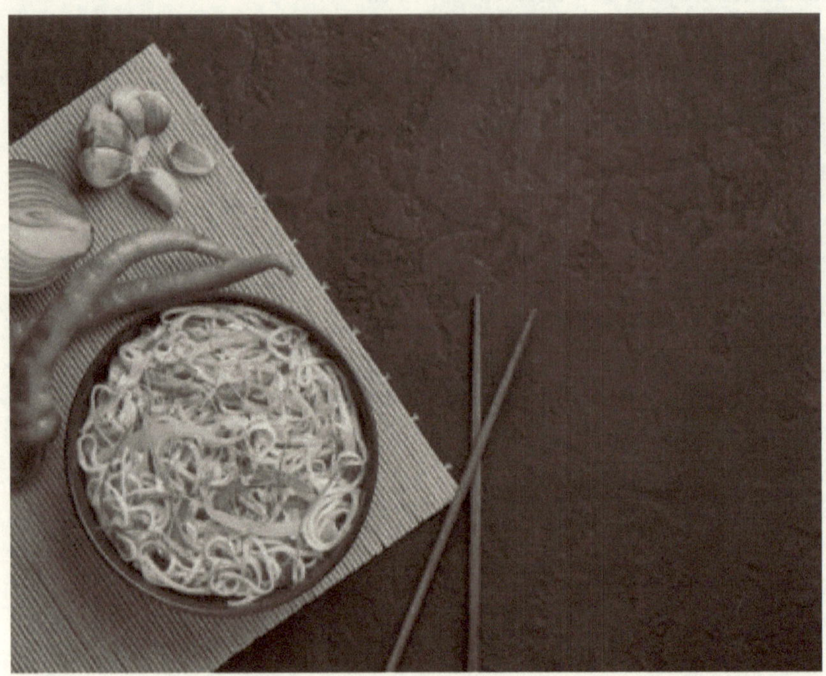

Serves: 6-8

Ingredients

2 tablespoons rice vinegar

¼ cup coconut sugar

¼ cup low sodium soy sauce

½ teaspoon red chili pepper flakes

7 medium cloves garlic, minced

1 cup sliced green onions, divided

1½ tablespoons toasted sesame oil

1 pound brown rice spaghetti

Sesame seeds for garnish

Directions

1. Over medium-low heat, heat a large pan and then pour in sesame oil.

2. Once warmed, stir in red chili flakes, garlic and green onions. Cook until the garlic is fragrant and light golden brown while stirring often.

3. Now add in rice vinegar, coconut sugar and soy sauce and stir to mix. Add in prepared and well drained noodles while tossing to coat them in the sauce.

4. Cook the noodles until heated through, in about 1-2 minutes or so.

5. Once done, garnish with a sprinkle of sesame seeds and the remaining sliced green onions. Serve the noodles instantly!

Snacks & Desserts Recipes

Blueberry Chia Jam Bars

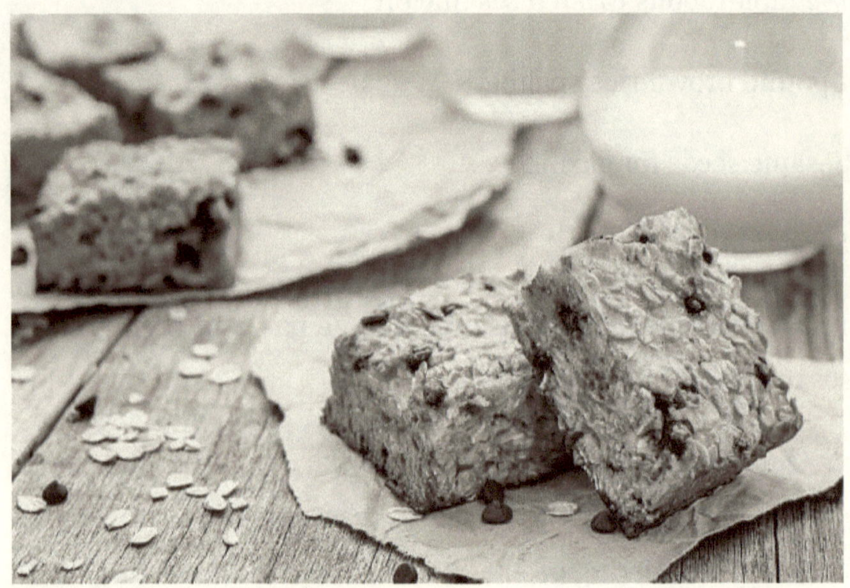

Serves: 16

Ingredients

1 teaspoon vanilla or almond extract

1/4 cup water

1/4 cup maple syrup

1 tablespoon chia seeds

1 1/2 cups gluten-free rolled oats

1 1/2 cups raw almonds

For Blueberry layer

2 tablespoons maple syrup

1/3 cup + 1 tablespoon chia seeds

12 oz. blueberries, fresh or frozen

Topping

1/3 cup maple syrup

1/3 cup coconut oil

1/3 cup cacao powder

Directions

1. Using unbleached parchment paper, line a 9 by 5 pan loaf and set aside. Put the main ingredients in a blender and pulse to combine.

2. Press the mixture evenly onto the parchment-lined pan using a spatula. Process the blueberries in a blender or food processor.

3. Add in chia seeds and puree to blend. Allow the mixture to sit until it thickens, for about 20 minutes. Then spread it over the pan-loaf ingredients.

4. Mix the topping ingredients in a small bowl and pour over the chia jam blueberry layer. Spread the topping evenly.

5. Now freeze to bars until firm then let thaw for 15-20 minutes at room temperature. Cut and serve or store the bars for up to a week in the fridge.

Blueberry Coconut Popsicles

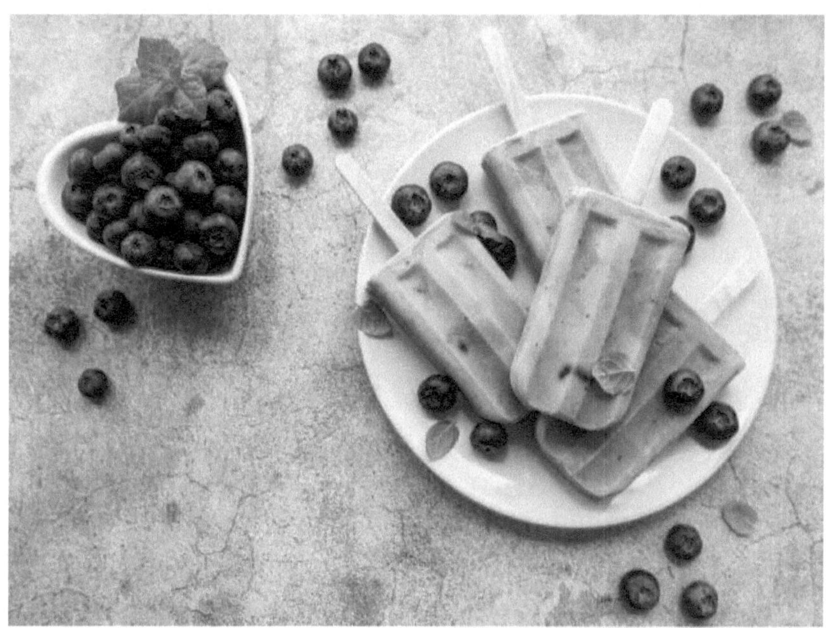

Serves: 10

Ingredients

2-3 tablespoons pure maple syrup

3 cups fresh blueberries

1 can full-fat coconut milk

Directions

1. To a blender, add maple syrup, blueberries and coconut milk and process until smooth. Scrap down the sides of the food processor as required.

2. Move the mixture into a Popsicle mold leaving around ¼ inch part at the top of the mold to help the popsicles expand in the freezer.

3. Follow the mold directions to insert the Popsicle sticks into the prepared mold. Freeze the Popsicle for about 6 to 8 hours.

4. Once hard enough, remove from the freezer and then let thaw for 1-2 minutes. You can run the mold lukewarm water to loosen the popsicles if need be.

5. Put the Popsicle mold on flat surface and gently wiggle the snack out. Serve!

Pineapple Coconut Black Ice Cream

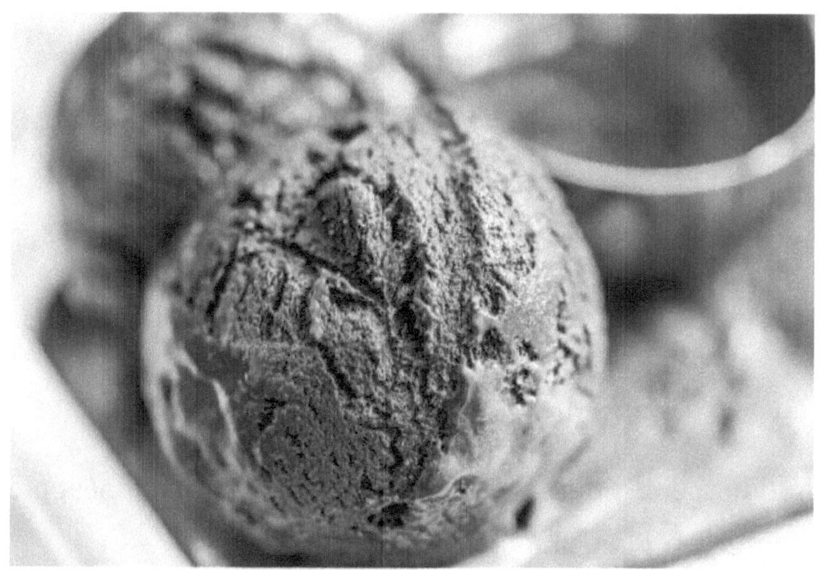

Serves: 6

Ingredients

3 ¼ tablespoon activated black charcoal

Small pinch of salt

1 teaspoon coconut extract

1 teaspoon vanilla extract

¾ cup white sugar

½ cup almond milk

1 cup crushed pineapple

1 cup raw cashews, soaked 2 days and rinsed

2 cups full fat coconut milk, chilled

Directions

1. Mix together almond milk and cashews in a high speed blender to obtain a thick and creamy consistency.

2. Add in the rest of the ingredients apart from the pineapple and puree to obtain smooth creamy.

3. Move the ice cream to a bowl and whisk in pineapple and mix well. Add the mixture to the ice cream maker and follow the manufacturer's instructions to churn.

4. As soon as you obtain creamy frozen ice cream, serve or store in airtight container. Keep it chilled for at least 2 hours to freeze fully.

Turmeric Cauliflower Puree

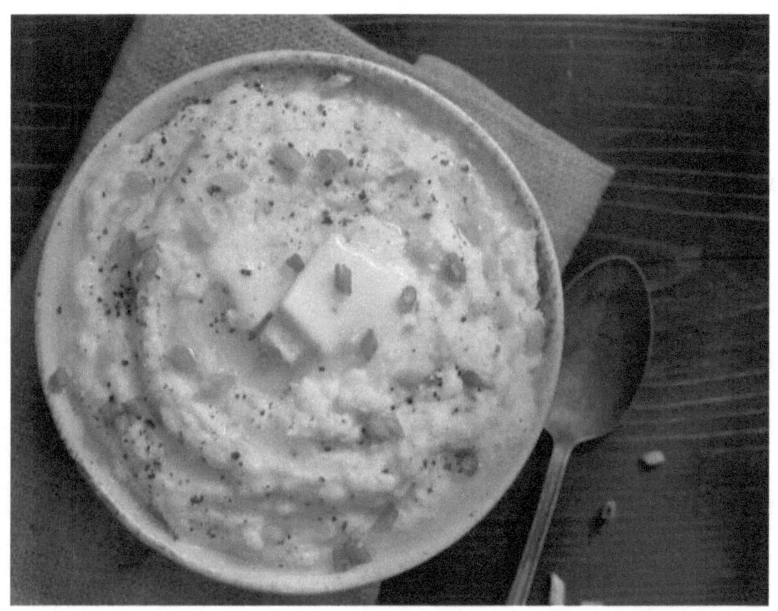

Serves 1

Ingredients

Juice of 1 fresh lemon

2 tablespoons nutritional yeast, optional

2 cups veggie broth

3 cups steamed cauliflower

1 clove garlic

1 15 ounce can white beans, drained

1 teaspoon turmeric powder

1/2 teaspoon onion powder

1/4 cup raw cashews, soaked and drained

Salt, to taste

Pepper, to taste

Steamed cauliflower, for garnish

Directions

1. In a food processor or blender, puree the ingredients until smooth.

2. If using a high-speed blender, process for about 4-6 minutes to blend and heat the mixture simultaneously.

3. For regular blender, move the smooth puree to a pot and then warm it. Serve and enjoy.

Fresh Corn Salad

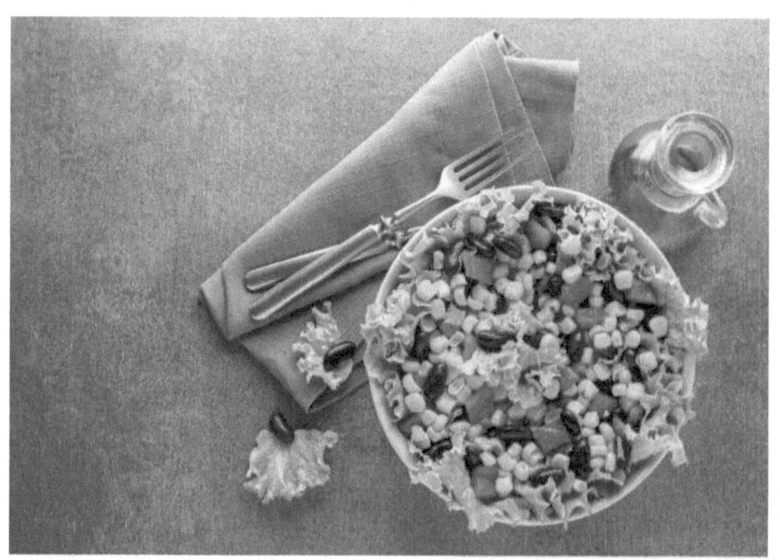

Serves 4 to 6

Ingredients

1/2 cup julicnncd fresh basil leaves

1/2 teaspoon black pepper, freshly ground

1/2 teaspoon kosher salt

3 tablespoons good olive oil

3 tablespoons cider vinegar

1/2 cup small-diced red onion

5 ears of corn, shucked

Directions

1. Cook the corn in a large pot that has boiling salted water until the starchiness is done, or for approximately 3 minutes.

2. Drain and then immerse the corn in ice water until cool. Then cut the kernels off the cob, while cutting close to the cob.

3. Toss the kernels in a bowl along with pepper, salt, olive oil, vinegar and red onions.

4. Then toss in fresh basil, taste and adjust the seasoning accordingly. Serve either warm or cold.

Crispy Kale Chips

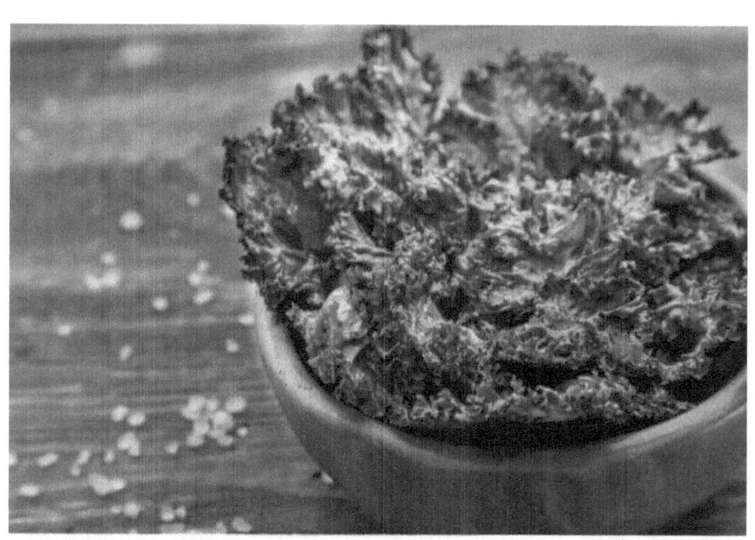

Serves: 8

Ingredients

2 tablespoons filtered water

½ teaspoon gray sea salt or pink rock salt

1 tablespoon raw honey

2 tablespoons nutritional yeast

1 lemon, juiced

1 cup sweet potato, grated

1 cup fresh cashews, soaked 2 hours

2 bunches green curly kales, cut into bite sizes

Directions

1. In a food processor or blender, process all the ingredients, apart from kales, until smooth.

2. Put the kale in a large mixing bowl and then pour over the blended ingredients. Combine fully with your hands so that to coat the kale.

3. Transfer the kale onto unbleached parchment paper, and then set the oven to 150 degrees to dehydrate the kales for 2 hours.

4. Turn the leaves at some point to ensure smooth drying. Once done, remove from the oven and keep into an airtight container.

Baked Onion Bhajis

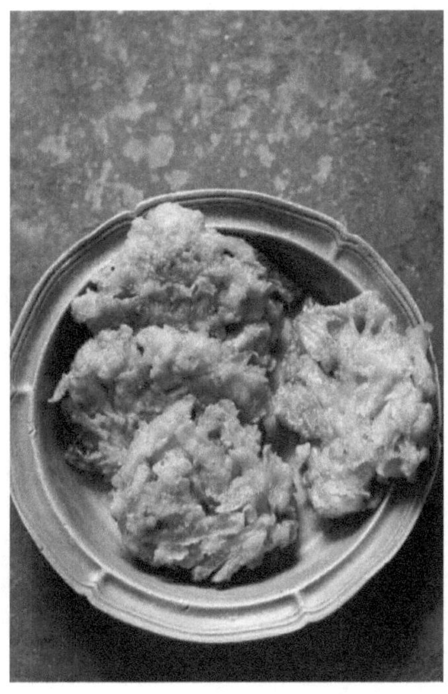

Serves: 8

Ingredients

1 tablespoon tomato puree

Extra-virgin olive oil, as needed

1/2 teaspoon coriander, ground

1/2 teaspoon cumin

1 pinch salt

5 tablespoons chickpea flour

5 small onions, sliced 5 mm thick

Enough water

For Spices

1/4 teaspoon chili powder

1/4 teaspoon ginger, ground

1/4 teaspoon cumin, ground

1/2 teaspoon coriander, ground

1/2 teaspoon turmeric, ground

Directions

1. First preheat your oven to 200 C; and then line a baking tray using baking parchment.

2. In a frying pan, sweat the onions with some oil for around 6-8 minutes, or until translucent.

3. Now sprinkle the chili powder and stir together, and follow with coriander, ginger, cumin and turmeric. Combine fully and remove from heat.

4. In a medium bowl, mix together coriander, salt, cumin and chickpea flour and then and in tomato puree and onions.

5. Add in a sufficient amount of water to achieve required consistency, to obtain a wet and easy to stir mixture.

6. Now drizzle oil on a tray and add 2 tablespoons of the onion mix for each bhaji. Use the back of the spoon to flatten it slightly.

7. In the preheated oven, bake on the middle shelf for around 20-25 minutes, and then drizzle some oil on top of the bhajis.

8. Bake for 25 more minutes to obtain a golden brown dish. Then serve and enjoy.

Cherry Chocolate Shake

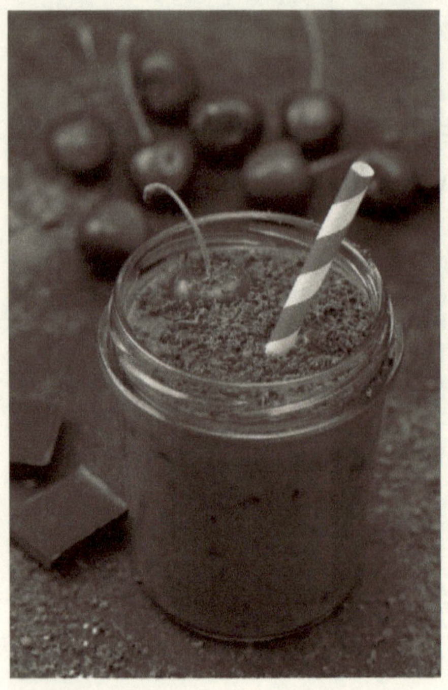

Serves 1

Ingredients

Ice cubes as desired

Few drops of liquid stevia

½ teaspoon pure vanilla extract

1 cup coconut; almond or flax milk

½ cup frozen dark cherries, pitted

1 tablespoon cocoa powder, unsweetened, unprocessed

Directions

1. In a blender, put all the ingredients and then process to smoothness.

2. Serve and enjoy.

Arctic Lime Freeze

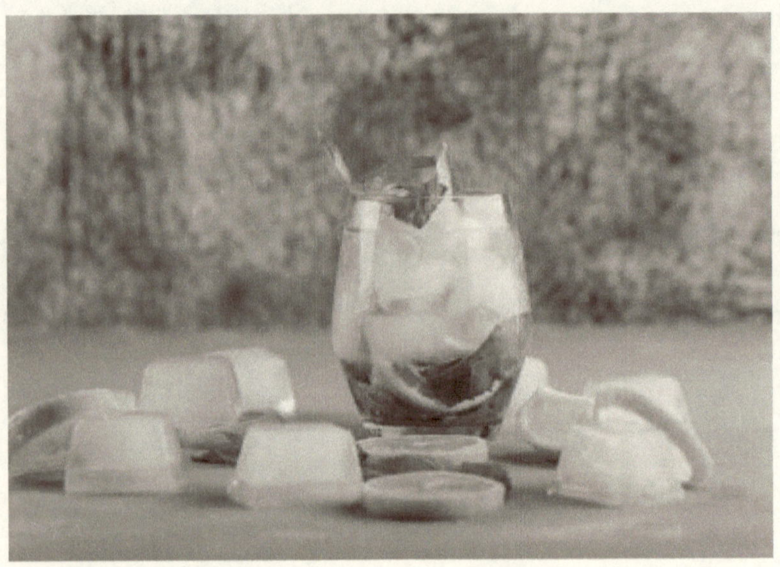

Serves 5

Ingredients

1 1/2 cups water

1 (12.3-ounce) package silken firm tofu, drained

1 (12-ounce) can thawed limeade concentrate, undiluted

Grated lime rind

Mint sprigs

Directions

1. Mix together tofu and limeade in a blender and puree until smooth. Add in water and pulse to incorporate.

2. Pour the ingredients into the freezer can of the ice-cream freezer and keep chilled.

3. Spoon into a freezer-safe bowl, cover and keep chilled for 2 hours.

4. Once firm enough garnish with mint and rind if you like.

Gluten-free Raspberry Shortcake

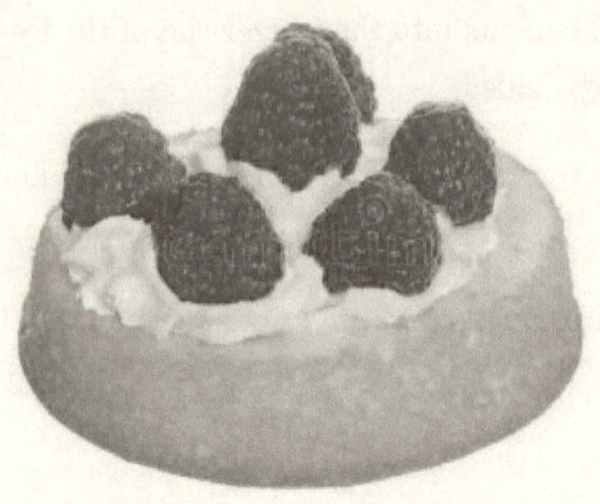

Serves 6

Ingredients

1/2 cup low-joule raspberry jam, melted

3 punnets raspberries

2 tablespoons icing sugar, sifted

1 teaspoon vanilla extract

500g low-fat ricotta

1 cup gluten-free vanilla soy milk

2 teaspoons baking powder, gluten-free

1/2 cup rice flour

3/4 cup desiccated coconut

3/4 cup skim milk powder

225g almond meal

Directions

1. Preheat the oven to 170 degrees F.

2. Then lightly coat a loose-bottomed 10 by 34 cm rectangular tart pan.

3. Mix together baking powder, rice flour, coconut, skim milk powder and almond meal in a bowl. Add in milk and stir to blend.

4. Press the batter into the tart pan and bake until golden and cooked through, in about 20-25 minutes. Let cool in the pan.

5. Now in a food processor, puree icing sugar, vanilla and the ricotta until smooth. Spread over the shortcake base and top with raspberries.

6. Brush the raspberries with melted jam, slice and serve the cake.

Life-Changing Loaf of Bread

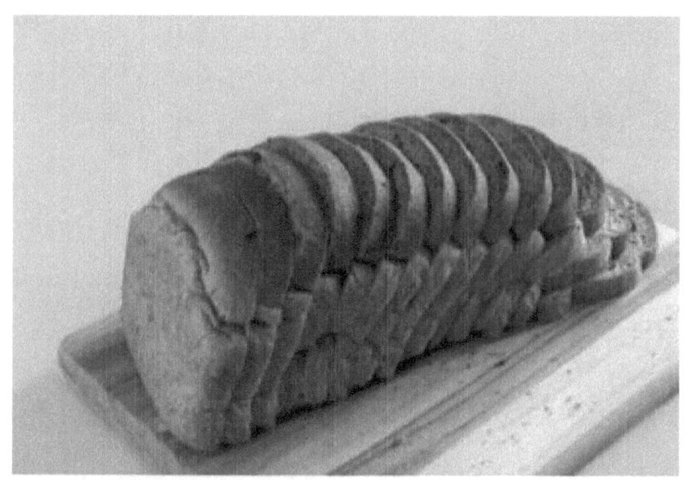

Yields: 1 loaf

Ingredients

1 1/2 cups water

3 tablespoons melted coconut oil or ghee

1 tablespoon maple syrup

1 teaspoon fine grain sea salt

4 tablespoons psyllium seed husks

2 tablespoons chia seeds

1 1/2 cups of rolled gluten-free oats

1/2 cup hazelnuts or almonds

1/2 cup flax seeds

1 cup sunflower seed kernels

Directions

1. Mix together all the dry ingredients in a parchment lined loaf pan and stir well.

2. Then whisk water, oil and maple syrup in a measuring cup. Add in the dry ingredients and combine well to blend fully to obtain very thick dough.

3. Using the back of a spoon, smooth out the dough then allow to rise all day or overnight. When done, it should retain its shape when you move the parchment.

4. Meanwhile, preheat your oven to 350 degrees F. Then put the loaf pan in the middle rack of the oven to bake for about 20 minutes.

5. Once cooked through, remove the bread from the pan loaf and put it upside down on the rack and bake for 30-40 minutes.

6. As soon as it sounds hollow when tapped, allow it to cool and then slice it. Store it in a tightly sealed container for a maximum for 5 days.

Coconut Cream Pie

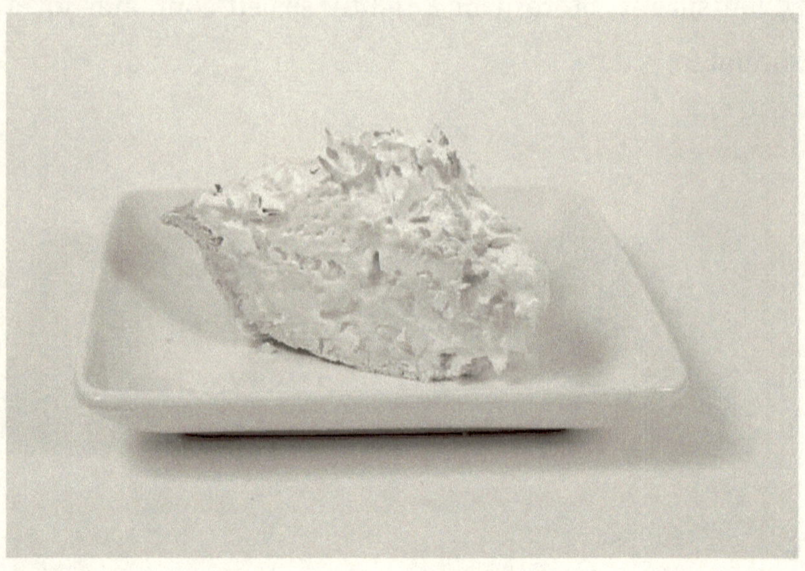

Serves 4

Ingredients

9-inch graham cracker crust

1 cup coconut, toasted

2 boxes vanilla pudding mix, fat-free

1 tablespoon coconut extract

2¾ cup skim milk

2 envelops Kraft dream topping whip, unprepared.

1 teaspoon coconut extract

Directions

1. Beat the whip topping mix, a cup of milk vanilla for 6 minutes on high heat until it turns very stiff.

2. Add the remaining milk, coconut extract and pudding mixes and beat on high for 2 minutes.

3. Fold the coconut as you pour in pie shell, and reserve 2 tablespoons of garnish if preferred.

4. Allow to cool for 4 hours and then sprinkle with the reserved coconut or fine chocolate curls.

5. Sprinkle lightly with low fat graham cracker crumbs (toasted).

Roasted Beet Dip

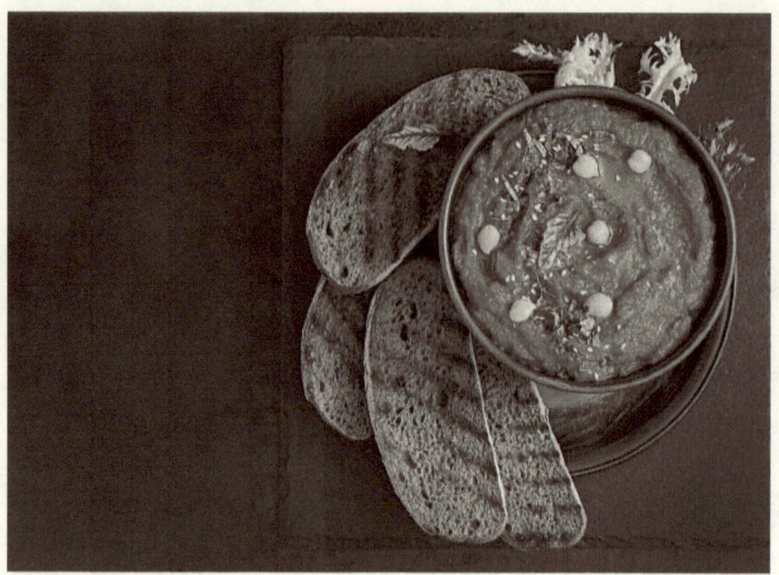

Serves: 2 Cups

Ingredients

1/3 cup loosely packed cilantro leaves, finely chopped

2 teaspoons fresh lemon juice

2 teaspoons green chile, chopped

2 teaspoons minced garlic

3/4 teaspoon coriander seeds

3/4 teaspoon cumin seeds

1/2 teaspoon Celtic sea salt

1/4 cup extra-virgin olive oil

4 cups peeled and cubed raw beets

Directions

1. Preheat your oven to 400 degrees F. Meanwhile, line a baking sheet with parchment paper or silicon liner.

2. Toss the beets with ¼ teaspoon of salt and 2 tablespoons. Then layer the beets on the baking sheet and roast for 1 hour. Toss occasionally, until the beets are tender.

3. In a heavy skillet, heat coriander and cumin over medium high heat for about 2 minutes, while stirring. Do not burn them, as they can develop bitterness.

4. Crush the seeds with a mortar and pestle grind in a spice grinder. Put the beets in a food processor and add in 2 tablespoons of oil, ¼ teaspoon salt, lemon juice, chile, garlic and the toasted and ground seeds.

5. Blast until fully incorporated then adjust the salt, lemon, chile and garlic to taste. Move the dip to a bowl and add in cilantro. Stir to mix and serve.

Beet Chocolate Pudding

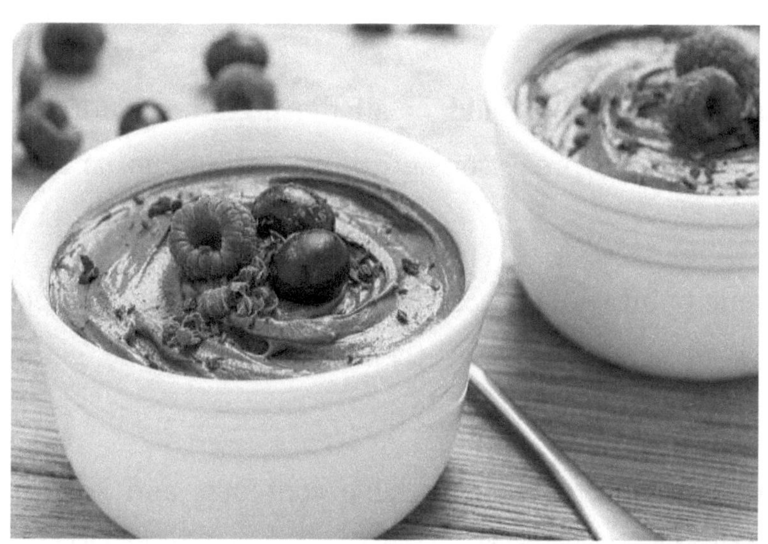

Serves: 4

Ingredients

1/8 teaspoon sea salt

1/2 teaspoon ground cinnamon

1/3 cup pure maple syrup

1/2 cup full-fat canned coconut milk

1/2 cup red beet roasted

1/2 cup unsweetened cocoa powder or raw cacao powder

2 large ripe avocados peeled and diced

Directions

1. To a food processor, add in all the ingredients for the pudding to a food processor and process to obtain smooth mixture.

2. At some point while processing, stop the blender a couple of times to scrap the sides then re-start again to get a smoother consistency.

3. Move the pudding to a sealable container and keep it chilled for a few hours. Serve it with coconut whipped cream.

Key Lime Pie

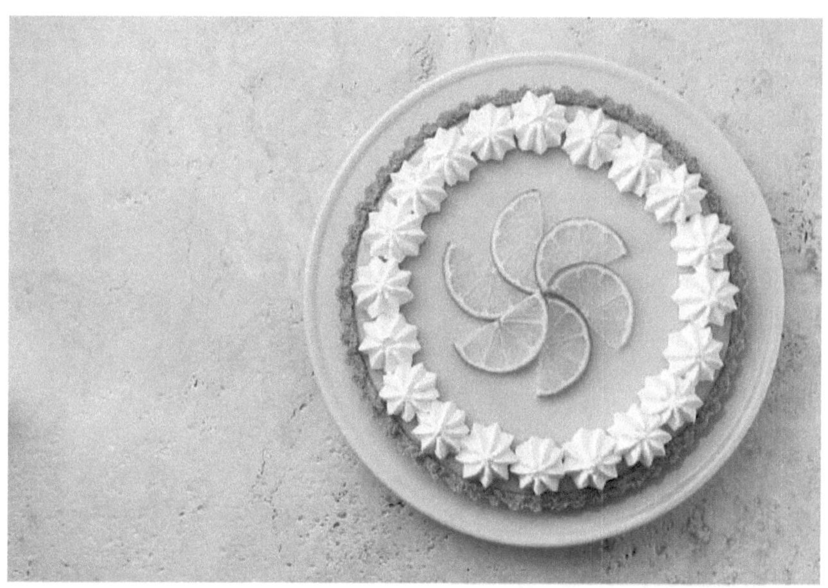

Servings: 8

For Crust

½ cup pitted Medjool dates

¼ teaspoon gray sea salt or pink rock salt

1 cup walnuts

1 cup shredded coconut, unsweetened

For Filling:

Kiwi or lime slices

Pinch of gray sea salt or pink rock salt

½ cup raw honey

1 teaspoon lime zest

3 tablespoons lime juice

3 firm avocados

Directions

1. In a food processor or blender, process walnuts, coconut and salt until it's coarsely ground.

2. Add in dates and process the mixture to achieve bread crumbs consistency or until the mixture starts to clump together.

3. Use a spoon or your fingers to press the mixture into the 9-inch pie plate and then put the crust in a freezer for around 15 minutes.

4. Now put the filling ingredients in a food processor and process to smoothness.

5. Once done, pour the fine mixture into the pie crust and then keep in the refrigerator for around 20 minutes.

6. Garnish with fresh kiwi or fresh slices or thin slices of lime if you like.

Turmeric Chia Pudding

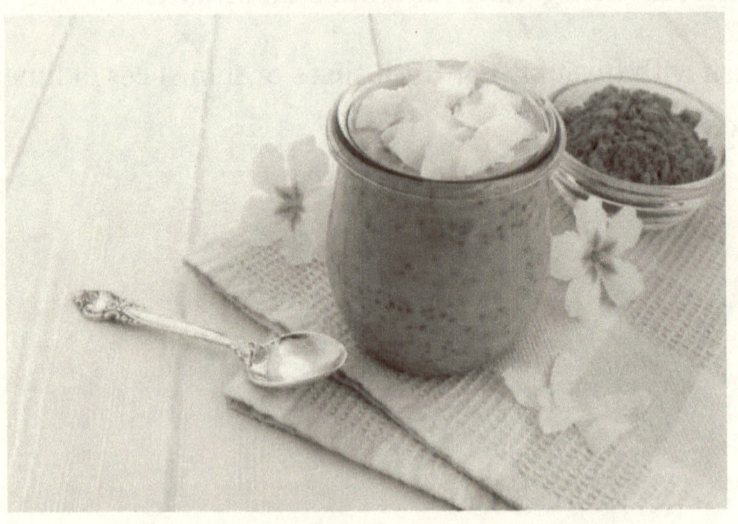

Serves: 2-4

Ingredients

⅛ teaspoon ground cloves

⅛ teaspoon ground cardamom

½ teaspoon cinnamon

1 teaspoon ground turmeric

2 tablespoons maple syrup

⅓ cup chia seeds

1 ½ cups cashew milk or almond milk

Directions

1. Combine together all the ingredients in a bowl.

2. Pour the mixture into individual jars or bowls then allow to set overnight.

3. Eat the pudding plain or top with nuts and fruits.

No doubt, preparing your own anti-inflammatory meals has never been simpler! You've got all you need as far as ideas on delicious meals are concerned. One challenge though, cooking your own meals requires ample time.

But in some cases, you may not have sufficient time to cook or you could be away from your house. So what should you do? Well, you can eat out but you must follow a few rules; otherwise, you could be making steps backward.

Tips for Eating Out

In cases where you need to eat out, you should observe this specific guideline: *carry foods with you!* Particularly, if going out for work or event, it's a good thing to carry a lunch bag that comprises of leftovers and snack foods, say almonds and dates.

Snacks like hummus, seeds, nuts and protein bars can help you ditch processed and sweet foods sold at your local restaurant. In special cases, you might carry your own ingredients into restaurants or other outdoor settings.

Ingredients such as herbs, spices, natural salad dressing, olive oil, lemon and avocado can be easily sneaked into your handbag. If visiting a restaurant, ask ahead if such practice is acceptable or if such products are served as part of the diet. If such arrangement fails, you can order a salad and later eat other foods at home.

Perhaps you can see the importance of making relevant lifestyle changes among them choosing how the foods you eat are cooked, right? Well, it doesn't just stop there. You should be aware that most life choices you make do have an indirect effect on levels of inflammatory responses and your general health too.

Here are a few ways you can further enhance your body's ability to combat chronic diseases arising from inflammation:

How To Deal With Inflammation Through Lifestyle Changes

Get sufficient sleep

Sleep is very important to your health. The process of your body resting and healing itself happens when you are sleeping. Research has shown that you need eight good hours of sleep in order to maintain a healthy body. It will probably shock you to know that inadequate sleep results to chronic inflammation. People who get insufficient sleep are known to produce high levels of inflammatory cytokines than those who get adequate sleep.

Peace of mind

Maintaining a peaceful mind is essential when you are fighting inflammation. Peace of mind helps you to stay away from stress, which if you let it, can worsen inflammatory symptoms. Stress normally activates adrenal glands, which in turn excrete stress hormones, which are adrenaline, cortisol, and noradrenaline. These hormones are amazing when it comes to soothing your stress but the ugly part is when your body goes under constant stress, which results, to the excessive production of the above hormones, which damages the tissues and causes inflammation. When this happens, your cells lose their sensitivity, which means they become less responsive and this will lead to inflammatory processes.

Sufficient hydration

Dehydration is your worst enemy when you are fighting inflammation. When you are dehydrated, your body turns into a multitude of reactions, which include inflammation. To avoid this, you must first understand that water is life then make a point of drinking 1-2 liters of water every day. You can also use lemon water, which has added alkalizing properties, which reduce inflammation.

You should make sure to take more water during hot weather or if you are pregnant or nursing. If you are already suffering from inflammation, you can try drinking lemon juice or water every morning since this has been shown to improve your condition in ways that you can't imagine.

Adequate physical activity

Involving yourself with regular physical activities has many benefits for your health. It helps you reduce inflammation, protects your muscles, heart and brain. All you need to do is to start with 5 minutes physical routines like press-ups, sit-ups, and crunches. You can combine these perfectly with your morning jog.

The regular exercises can boost your immune system and help you in preventing diseases, which normally result to cellular damages that lead to inflammation. So if you want to have a body that is free from inflammation, you will have to start exercising on a regular basis.

Stretching

Stretching is a fun way of dealing with inflammation. You can incorporate your stretching with deep breathing, which triggers positive chemical reactions in your body. Stretching reduces inflammation by mobilizing stored toxins that are found in your tissues making it easier for them to be deposited into your bloodstream, which disposes them safely.

Deep breathing

Breathing deeply activates your vagus nerve that goes on to encourage the release of acetylcholine, which turns off the inflammatory development in your body and this is why breathing is important in the fight against inflammation.

Relax

There is nothing as fulfilling as relaxing. When you have chronic stress or inflammation in your body, your best shot will be to find ways in which you can relax. Meditation and biofeedback therapies are two options that can be used to relax your mind and body. For instance, when you go for therapy, you are able to lay off all your burdens and this relaxes your entire body.

Techniques You Can Use To Reduce The Causes Of Inflammation

Make your environment as green as possible

You can reduce inflammation by taking care of your environment. You can do this by changing your life to a greener one. This means using natural cleaning products and natural detergents. Stay clear of air pollutants like fresheners and stop depending on dry cleaners. You can plant flowers in the house to cleanse the air for you.

Change your bad habits

There are a couple of bad habits, which encourage the process of inflammation. These habits include alcoholism, smoking cigarette, marijuana, and regular intake of caffeinated beverages. If you want to reduce inflammation, you must stop smoking and relying on stimulants. If quitting all by yourself seems hard, you can look for support groups in your area, which you can go and open up. The change in behavior will help to reduce inflammation as we have seen above.

Detoxification

It is almost impossible for you to escape the unhealthiness of our environment. Environmental toxins can really wear you off so you need to detoxify almost after every month. Detox is meant for cleansing your internal body to eliminate the risk of inflammation in your body.

Mind body treatments

Using medication and steroids works perfectly when soothing pain caused by inflammation but there is one tiny problem; the long term effects of the drugs can be lethal to your health and that is where mind body treatments come in as a better alternative. Massage, water therapy, and acupuncture are some natural examples of how you can deal with your pain.

Conclusion

I hope this book was able to help you to fight inflammation. I believe this book has been informative as well as educative to you. You have now known how inflammation affects your health and the different diseases that it can cause. Now you have all the information you need to fight inflammation by avoiding the foods that trigger inflammation as well as taking foods that fight inflammation. The book also provided some helpful ideas on some lifestyle changes you should make to fight inflammation so you have all you need to deal with inflammation.

Now is your turn to take action!

PS: I'd like your feedback. If you are happy with this book, please leave a review on Amazon.

Please leave a review for this book on Amazon by visiting the page below:

https://amzn.to/2VMR5qr